OUT OF THE ORDINARY

Out of the Ordinary

A LIFE OF GENDER AND SPIRITUAL TRANSITIONS

MICHAEL DILLON / LOBZANG JIVAKA

Edited and with an Introduction by
Jacob Lau and Cameron Partridge

FORDHAM UNIVERSITY PRESS

New York 2017

Fordham University Press has no responsibility for the
persistence or accuracy of URLs for external or third-party
Internet websites referred to in this publication and does
not guarantee that any content on such websites is, or will
remain, accurate or appropriate.

Fordham University Press also publishes its books in a
variety of electronic formats. Some content that appears in
print may not be available in electronic books.

Visit us online at www.fordhampress.com.

Library of Congress Cataloging-in-Publication Data
available online at http://catalog.loc.gov.

Printed in the United States of America
19 18 17   5 4 3 2 1
First edition

CONTENTS

Foreword by Susan Stryker   vii

Editors' Note   xi

"In His Own Way, In His Own Time":
An Introduction to *Out of the Ordinary*   1

Out of the Ordinary   27

Author's Introduction   29

Part I. Conquest of the Body

1. Birth and Origins   35
2. The Nursery   43
3. Schooldays   58
4. Oxford   74
5. War—The Darkest of Days   88

Part II. Conquest of the Mind

6. Medical Student   109
7. Resident Medical Officer   131
8. Surgeon M.N.   142
9. On the Haj   155
10. Round the World   168
11. Interlude Ashore   187
12. The Last Voyage   202
13. *Imji Getsul*   223

Michael Dillon / Lobzang Jivaka: A Timeline   233

Acknowledgments   237

Susan Stryker

More than twenty-five years ago, when I first started seriously researching transgender history, I came across an anecdote in Liz Hodgkinson's 1989 biography, *Michael née Laura: The World's First Female to Male Transsexual,* about an unpublished manuscript that whetted my curiosity. Hodgkinson's book recounted the life of a person whom she called Michael Dillon, who had been given the name Laura Maude Dillon at birth in 1915 and who would die soon after taking the additional name of Lobzang Jivaka in 1962. The manuscript in question was an autobiography that recounted this man's remarkable life, completed mere days before his untimely death.

Dillon, or Jivaka, as you will discover in the pages that follow, was a fascinating fellow—not, in truth, the first female-to-male transsexual but almost certainly the first to have undergone phalloplasty (the surgical construction of a penis) in a series of procedures carried out in the late 1940s, after having started taking testosterone a few years earlier. He was an insatiably inquisitive, doggedly determined person whose quest to actualize his sense of self led him not only to transition from social womanhood to life as a man but to attend university at Oxford, become a doctor, serve as a shipboard medical officer sailing the seven seas, read widely in various religious and spiritual traditions, and eventually to take vows as a novitiate monk in a Buddhist monastery. He was a minor member of the British aristocracy, to boot.

While still a medical student in the midst of gender transition in 1946, Dillon authored an obscure but erudite little book, *Self: An Essay on Ethics and Endocrinology,* which functioned as cryptoautobiography. Grounded in his self-experimentation with hormones but written in an impersonal voice in spite of his deeply personal, embodied stake in the argument, it laid out, from the perspective of sexological science, a cogent case for the ethical use of medical procedures to change the sex-signifying characteristics of people like himself who experienced a mismatch between their inner and outer realities. Seen through a contemporary transgender lens, *Self* is a prescient account, *avant la lettre,* of the "transsexual discourse" that took shape in the mid–twentieth century. It is a tale told by one of the first individuals to comprehend the possibility of using the plastic surgeries developed to repair the combat-injured genitals of male soldiers and the hormones synthesized in the hope of extending life or restoring the libido's lost vigor for the novel purpose of "changing sex." Although Dr. Harry Benjamin is generally credited with developing the "logic of treatment" for transsexual medical care in his 1966 book *The Transsexual Phenomenon*, Dillon actually got there first, a full two decades earlier.

As a young transgender historian searching for kindred spirits a quarter-century ago, Dillon's *Self* left me hungering for a fuller, first-person perspective on Dillon's self—something a biography might describe but by definition could never get inside of. Sadly, Dillon's published first-person writings—a slender 1957 volume, *Poems of Truth*, and Jivaka's 1962 *Imji Getsul: An English Buddhist in a Tibetan Monastery*—are woefully short on subjective, introspective detail. Hence the romantic allure for me over the decades of his unpublished autobiographical manuscript—it functioned as a vague receptacle that held half-formed fantasies about connecting with a lost and disremembered past—and my great delight, all these many years later, at being asked to write a foreword to that autobiography, now that it is finally seeing print.

Dillon/Jivaka's *Out of the Ordinary* long remained unpublished, but it was never lost. The manuscript, bearing both of the author's names, was mailed from India shortly before the author's death, and it arrived on the desk of the literary agent John Johnson shortly after the author's death. Dillon/Jivaka's transphobic and publicity-averse brother—Sir Robert Dillon, eighth Baronet of Lismullen—wished the manuscript destroyed; Johnson nevertheless pursued posthumous publication, without success, though whether because the work was deemed to lack literary merit or commercial potential or from publishers' fears of a lawsuit by the family remains unclear. Johnson's successor at the literary agency, Andrew Hewson, retained a copy of the manuscript, which he made available to Liz Hodgkinson in the 1980s. Indeed, *Out of the Ordinary* was a crucial source for Hodgkinson's *Michael née Laura*, though she trod lightly around the fact, lest the uncooperative and hostile Dillon family continue to seek the manuscript's destruction.

Two decades later, Hewson made the manuscript available to another researcher, Pagan Kennedy, who was working on her own biography of Dillon/Jivaka, *The First Man-Made Man*, published in 2007. At a bookstore reading in Brookline, Massachusetts, that year, Kennedy mentioned *Out of the Ordinary* and the fact that it remained unpublished. Two young trans* scholars from the Harvard Divinity School, Cameron Partridge and Jacob Lau, were in the audience that night. They approached Kennedy, who made her digital photographs of the manuscript available to them, and the result is the book you now hold in your hands.

Reading *Out of the Ordinary* at long last, it feels too constraining to characterize the book as primarily a "transsexual autobiography," too partial to foreground the author's being "the first manmade man" or "the first female-to-male transsexual." First and foremost, the author of this text was a seeker after truth who traveled wherever his queries led him. His peregrinations from Laura to Michael to Lobzang were all of a piece, as spiritual and metaphysical as they were intellectual and transsexual and medical. We tend to privilege a materialist scientific epistemology in the modern secular West and in doing so easily fall into apprehending Dillon first and foremost as a certain kind of being called a transsexual who also happened to have a mystical bent. It's harder to appreciate that the discourse of transsexuality produces one kind of truth-effect, and religious seeking another, and that Dillon's becoming-Jivaka was an embrace of both as well as a refusal to put one "technology of the self" above the other.

If the question "Who am I?" is, for all of us, as Winston Churchill once said of Russia, "a riddle, wrapped in a mystery, inside an enigma," Dillon/ Jivaka's pursuit of his own particular answer to that conundrum took him to the primal scene of meaning making, where we seem to discern something ineffable moving against the veil of representation. This *topos* of ontological construction is the place creation myths come from, and revelations, as well as the veridictions of science; it all depends on how the experience of that encounter is framed, narrated, validated, and transmitted. In their introduction to *Out of the Ordinary*, Partridge and Lau, both students of religion, are especially attuned to this dual dimension of Dillon/ Jivaka's life quest and consequently deepen our understanding of him— and of the nonsecular qualities that transsexual/transgender life processes can harbor.

So much has changed since the early 1990s, when I discovered Lobzang née Michael née Laura's story through Liz Hodgkinson's exemplary biographical research and first caught a glimpse of the manuscript that became this book. "Transgender" has exploded in the intervening years. It is no longer an obscure and virtually unknown topic, one of greatest interest to transgender people themselves. It currently saturates mass media on a daily basis and is the subject of widespread attention, fascination, consternation, and concern. Transgender studies has emerged since then as an interdisciplinary academic specialization in its own right, in which knowledge of trans* lives and histories is being produced not just by medical and legal authorities but from any number of viewpoints, including those of trans* people themselves.

But much remains the same. Struggles over the reality of trans* people's gender identifications and over the means through which we make those identifications discernable through the actions of our flesh still lie at the heart of the violence, marginalization, stigmatization, and discrimination we are far too often made to suffer. *Out of the Ordinary* tells the story of a remarkable life, and it should find an eager readership in our transgender-obsessed contemporary culture, among transgender and cisgender people alike. It provides welcome empirical content for trans* studies scholars seeking more information about the conditions of life for trans* people in the mid–twentieth century. But it attests as well to something greater: the fierce will to make real for others the inner reality that trans* people experience of themselves. That capacity to transform one reality into another is something trans* people often discover within themselves for the sake of their own survival; it is our gift to others to bear witness to the fact that this is a capacity within us all. That's a lesson Dillon/Jivaka learned more than half a century ago and one he can still teach us today.

Out of the Ordinary was typewritten on onionskin paper with sparse hand-written edits. We have transcribed the memoir from digital photographs and photocopies of the original onionskin that were generously provided to us by Pagan Kennedy. In an effort to preserve Dillon/Jivaka's intended phrasing we have largely integrated his edits into the body of the text without noting them. Occasionally, when we felt that the raw, layered quality of the handwritten notes was important to preserve, we shared them as footnotes so that the reader can see them on the page in quotations. In one case, a handwritten note appears not in a footnote but at the end of the final chapter. It indicates that the entire final chapter was tentative and could be scrapped depending on whether the author's history of transition had been definitively revealed before the memoir's publication. We felt it important to preserve that note as part of the historical record.

Otherwise, we used sparse notes to point the reader to historical context, to spell out acronyms, or to explain references that may be confusing.

OUT OF THE ORDINARY

"In His Own Way, In His Own Time":
An Introduction to *Out of the Ordinary*

Jacob Lau and Cameron Partridge

On May 15, 1962, the Tibetan Buddhist monastic novice Lobzang Jivaka (1915–1962) died in the Civil Hospital of Dalhousie in the Punjab region of India after collapsing on a remote mountain pass.[1] Only days before on his forty-seventh birthday, he had mailed his just-finished memoir entitled *Out of the Ordinary* to his literary agent in London. Typed beneath his Buddhist name on the title page was the British Christian name in which he had reregistered in 1943, Michael Dillon.[2] "Dr. Dillon felt there was no reason why, finally, his story could not be told," the agent, John Johnson, later stated to the *Sunday Telegraph*. "He wanted to tell it in his own way, in his own time."[3]

Dillon/Jivaka—as we refer to his textual authorship out of respect for the names he claimed on that title page[4]—had good reason for wanting to narrate his life on his own terms. As a man who had been assigned female at birth, having transitioned between 1939 and 1949, he had been on guard against media exposure for decades. From the years of his transition into the mid-1950s, a plethora of "sex change" stories had hit the headlines, telling of Roberta Cowell, Christine Jorgensen ("Ex-GI Becomes Blond Beauty," the *New York Daily News* trumpeted on December 1st, 1952), Dr. Ewan

Forbes ("The Sex Change," as *Man's Day* magazine reported c. 1953), Michael Harford, and Robert Allen.[5] Dillon/Jivaka rejected both the stories and their terminology.[6] Deeply concerned about privacy, he fundamentally distrusted what non-gender-variant people might do with such accounts. Indeed, the 1958 exposure of his own history while he served as a ship's surgeon in the British Merchant Navy traumatized him enough that he left his ship in India to immerse himself in Buddhist monastic life, "renouncing the world," as he referred to it. Even in India, the threat of his past undoing his new life emerged as a catalyst for change: this time, a decision to tell his story himself.

Faced with the possibility that a fellow British Buddhist monk, Urgyen Sangharakshita, was preparing to reveal his history in a respected Buddhist journal, Dillon/Jivaka decided to try to beat him to the punch.[7] As Pagan Kennedy has shown in her 2007 book *The First Man-Made Man*, Dillon/Jivaka wrote to Sangharakshita, requesting that he send the large envelope containing the memoir, composed with the aid of detailed journals.[8] Upon receiving the envelope, Dillon/Jivaka added the last chapter and a Foreword (which we refer to in this volume as the Author's Introduction). He then lightly edited his manuscript with marginal notations and put it in the mail. Within days he would be dead. Although he had suffered several illnesses, aided by chronic malnourishment in India, his death was sudden and unexpected. Some even wondered if he had been poisoned.[9] So soon did he die after mailing the manuscript that news of his death reached his agent John Johnson ahead of the memoir, and indeed the manuscript's arrival came as quite a surprise.[10]

Despite the dramatic story unfolding within its pages and behind its emergence, the memoir did not come out and in fact has never been published before now. Reasons for this failure are numerous, overlapping, and difficult to pin down. Dillon's will seems to have been either disputed or not acknowledged. His one sibling, a brother, Robert, who was the heir to a minor aristocratic title (the Baronet of Lismullen, to which Dillon/Jivaka was next in line because his brother had no children), did not want to be associated with news of his brother's transition.[11] One obituary even reported that Robert wanted the manuscript burned.[12] Dillon/Jivaka's writing style, which at points can be stiff and didactic, may also have been viewed as a stumbling block to publication. Then again, perhaps publishers did not take Dillon/Jivaka's story seriously because of a perceived greater public interest in—and often transmisogynistic objectification of—transgender women.[13] Perhaps the truth is some combination of the above.

Whatever the reason, that the memoir has thus far remained unpublished has been a loss to multiple readerships, not least to an increasingly empowered transgender community eager to engage with the historical sources of its pioneers. Indeed, because the memoir is composed under both his Christian and Buddhist names, it would have rendered Dillon/Jivaka, as Jamison Green might put it, "a visible man."[14] As Pagan Kennedy has noted, not only would he have become one of the first men to be open about his history of transition, had he lived, but even in death, he "might have offered a model [for such openness], if his book had appeared in print."[15] Although both Liz Hodgkinson and Kennedy[16] draw upon and, thankfully, reveal the existence of the memoir in their respective studies of Dillon/Jivaka, the fullness of the author's own narrative embodiment, as Jay Prosser might put it, has remained out of sight, interred in a London warehouse for half a century.[17]

We now return to that narrative body, disinterring it out of a desire to honor Dillon/Jivaka's own wishes and to enable his various constituencies—from grassroots transgender communities to scholars of trans, queer, and postcolonial studies, including their intersections with the study of religion in general and of Buddhism in particular, with the history of science and other scholarly disciplines—to engage directly with a fuller measure of his writings. It is high time, we believe, for this work to take its rightful place in the growing body of literature of and about transsexual and transgender people.[18]

A Life Characterized by Change

Born May 1, 1915, in Ladbroke Grove in the London borough of Kensington, Dillon was named after his mother, Laura Maude, who died between six and ten days after giving birth.[19] Dillon's father, Robert Dillon, struggled with alcoholism and left the raising of Michael and his older brother Bobby to their maiden aunts before dying of pneumonia when Dillon was ten.[20] From the very start, the memoir emphasizes the role of religion in his upbringing. His description of being raised in the Church of England features not so much his experience of church services or the devotion of his aunts (which he critiques as rote) as the mentorship he received from successive vicars. He speaks fondly of the Rev. C. S. T. Watkins, for whom he expressed a "hero-worship." Indeed, the Reverend Watkins seems to have helped open the door to theological reflection for the young Dillon:

After my period with Tarzan of the Apes had exhausted itself from
sheer rereading and had been manifested by a prolonged effort to
develop my muscles by all kinds of exercises and extra time spent in the
gymnasium . . . I turned, under the influence of my hero-worship of the
Vicar to books on theology.

But this was not wholly due to the Vicar's presence. For a year past
there had been stirrings in my mind of a curious nature which no one
seemed able to understand if I tried to talk about them. The utter
uselessness of the lives of the aunts and of their friends was puzzling
me and causing me to ask the question: what is the purpose of life?
What are we here for? And very soon it became specifically: what is
the purpose of my life? And shortly afterwards I was contemplating the
problem of what one had done to justify one's existence if one was on
the point of death. This was to be the first sign of that driving desire
to know which was going to pursue me for the rest of my life. In a few
years I was calling it the Search for Truth and it went through many
vicissitudes before I found myself anywhere near an answer.[21]

The vicar influenced Dillon not to take his own tradition at face value but
to delve into it, using his intellectual gifts to wrestle with his deepest questions. This habit of intellectual-spiritual inquiry became a lifelong practice
for Dillon, one that would take him beyond the boundaries of Christianity and into the esoteric spiritual writings of P. D. Ouspensky and G. I.
Gurdjieff, into dialogue with Tuesday Lobsang Rampa, and ultimately into
Theravada and Mahayana Buddhism.

This journey unfolded in several stages, initially moving from childhood
in Folkestone, England, to university at Oxford, the Reverend Watkins's
alma mater. Dillon's Oxford years come across as fraught with the tensions
of building crises of gender and vocation but at the same time as a source
of lifelong nostalgia. Indeed, one of the few biographical details Jivaka al-
lows in his most well-known book *Imji Getsul* is his identity as "Oxford
Man," a moniker he could only claim in retrospect, since he had attended a
women's college while there. Early on at Oxford, Dillon studied theology
but switched to classics (or "Greats," as it is called there) once he was convinced that becoming an Anglican deaconess was not a suitable vocation.
He also took up rowing with great vigor during these years, seeking to put
women's teams on the map. During this time, both gender and sexuality
became sources of personal consternation for him. He donned an Eton
crop, rode a motorcycle, smoked a pipe, and confided in trusted comrades
about his attraction to women. How did Dillon make sense of these experiences and desires?

Here the memoir not only narrates Dillon's young adult struggles, not only indicates a confusing haze of terminology at the intersection of what contemporary "Western" readers would call gender and sexuality (or, even more specifically, gender identity and its expression and sexual orientation), but also and perhaps most importantly reveals how the forty-seven-year-old Dillon associated his own life with the identity terms available to him. Some he engaged with, others he avoided. Comrades termed him "probably homosexual," and while he confesses having no evidence to the contrary, he never claims the label with any enthusiasm. Before long, both in his life and text, the term simply drops out, never to be replaced. The English term "transsexual" had not yet been coined when Dillon began embarking upon and writing about transition and, by the time of the memoir's composition, he either had not heard it or (as with the language of "sex change") deliberately eschewed it.

Uncharted Territory

Dillon's immediate postcollege years were particularly difficult. Not only was World War II starting up, but reactions by prospective employers to what would now be termed his gender expression—again, his haircut, dress, and general outward manner—were also creating barriers to his steady employment. Added to this was his growing sense that he needed to do something about his inner turmoil. In the absence of any obvious solutions, he sought out help from a local doctor.

> Somehow I heard of a doctor in the town who was said to be an expert on sex problems and to him I went to seek advice. He was interested and wished to help, at first postulating that a psychiatrist friend of his be brought in to make it an official experiment. So to the psychiatrist I went in all good faith and answered all his questions but the next time I visited the doctor full of hope he had suddenly become afraid and, expecting his own call-up shortly, which might mean leaving me in a half-finished and worse state than before, he backed out and I rode back to my digs once more in gloom, but in my pocket were some male hormone tablets he had thrown across the table to me. "See what they can do," he had said.[22]

This rollercoaster of emotion—openness, optimism, good faith, and gloom —would be followed by anger and a sense of betrayal when the psychiatrist shared his client's story with a doctor who turned out to work in the laboratory where Dillon had landed a job. When his workmates began joking,

"Miss Dillon wants to become a man!" he left.[23] After that, the only place he could find work was in a garage, where the boss hired him despite "not [being] sure," as Dillon/Jivaka puts it, "what to make of someone whose skirt belied the upper half."[24] There his workmates wasted no time in telling all newcomers, "you see that fellow over there? Well, he's not a man he's a girl."[25] Even the workshop foreman, "whose ear drums had been burst in the Great War and who had to have everything written down for him, had had this written too."[26] Of these "four miserable years," Dillon/Jivaka would add by hand, then cross out: "It was the worst period of my life."[27]

In the absence of any connection—medical, workplace, social—to other cross-gender-identified people, Dillon/Jivaka simply felt his way forward in the dark. Meanwhile, he seems to have had no initial idea just how significant were the tablets so casually tossed his way. Testosterone had been synthesized by a Dutch team only about four years earlier, in 1935.[28] From this point on, Dillon would self-administer the hormone, a regimen of which must be taken for life by those who wish to maintain its effects (now most often self-administered via shots, patches, or gels, under the care of an endocrinologist or primary care physician). Bodily changes would have appeared gradually, impacted as well by genetic predisposition: deepened voice, facial hair, increased muscle mass, a shift in the location of body fat, male-pattern baldness. Indeed, the rigorous manual labor of the garage was aided, he reports, "by the hormone tablets which I continued to take and which began to make my beard grow."[29] After a year, he continues, "the first step was taken—although it did not seem so at the time."[30] The few such comments suggest that Dillon happily learned about the effects of testosterone as they took place in his own body. Several years later, when newer acquaintances only knew him as male, "the relief was indescribable."[31]

Meanwhile, between his transition, hostile work environment, and the sheer intensity of fire watching after German raids (a civil defense task in which Dillon participated), Dillon applied his acute intellectual ability to the nascent field of sexology, focusing on the study of hormones, of homosexuality, and of intersexuality. The fruit of this labor was not only a greater sense of empowerment but also his first book, *Self: A Study in Ethics and Endocrinology*. This project also gave him a new vocational focus: he would become a medical doctor.[32] While many consider Harry Benjamin's *The Transsexual Phenomenon*[33] to be the first psychomedical work to define the concept of transsexuality as distinct from homosexuality, Hodgkinson, Kennedy, Hausman, Prosser, Meyerowitz, and Rubin all point out that

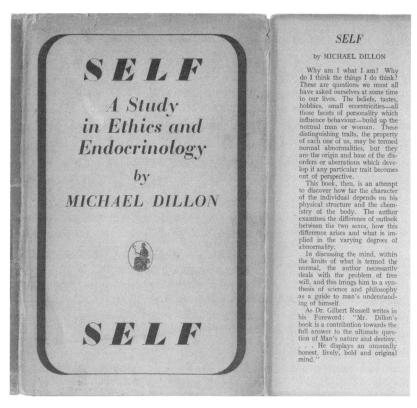

SELF

A Study in Ethics and Endocrinology

by

MICHAEL DILLON

SELF

SELF

by MICHAEL DILLON

Why am I what I am? Why do I think the things I do think? These are questions we must all have asked ourselves at some time in our lives. The beliefs, tastes, hobbies, small eccentricities—all those facets of personality which influence behaviour—build up the normal man or woman. These distinguishing traits, the property of each one of us, may be termed normal abnormalities, but they are the origin and base of the disorders or aberrations which develop if any particular trait becomes out of perspective.

This book, then, is an attempt to discover how far the character of the individual depends on his physical structure and the chemistry of the body. The author examines the difference of outlook between the two sexes, how this difference arises and what is implied in the varying degrees of abnormality.

In discussing the mind, within the limits of what is termed the normal, the author necessarily deals with the problem of free will, and this brings him to a synthesis of science and philosophy as a guide to man's understanding of himself.

As Dr. Gilbert Russell writes in his Foreword: "Mr. Dillon's book is a contribution towards the full answer to the ultimate question of Man's nature and destiny. . . . He displays an unusually honest, lively, bold and original mind."

Book jacket of *Self: A Study in Ethics and Endocrinology*, by Michael Dillon, 1946. *Self* was the first published work on the ethics of gender transition as distinct from homosexuality, written while the author was completing medical school.

the less widely distributed *Self* began to chart this territory twenty years earlier.

Writing *Out of the Ordinary* at a remove of several decades, Dillon / Jivaka depicts his transition within the frame of an ongoing process of transformation—or as he often terms it, "evolution." On the one hand, Dillon deeply engaged himself in the process of his transformation by reading everything he could find about medical interventions into sexual difference. On the other hand, he obtained the several surgical interventions he later underwent, like the testosterone pills themselves, almost by happenstance. Throughout his life, he appears to have suffered from bouts of hypoglycemia that caused him to pass out on occasion. More than once he reports landing in the hospital, where the challenge of being placed in gender-segregated wards actually helped connect Dillon with sympathetic care. An unnamed plastic surgeon in the second such instance, three years after Dillon began taking testosterone, suggested he get a double mastectomy and reregister as male (the U.S. equivalent of changing one's birth certificate).³⁴ Having studied with the renowned Dr. Harold Gillies, this surgeon referred Dillon to his teacher for a phalloplasty, the first of its kind performed for a patient assigned female at birth. The first of these thirteen operations was "the one thing of supreme importance" that took place in the summer of 1945,³⁵ Dillon/Jivaka recalls. With his coauthor Ralph Millard, Gillies later reported this intervention in the case study "Female with Male Outlook" in the 1957 book *The Principles and Art of Plastic Surgery*.³⁶

At Sea

After graduating from the medical school at Trinity College, Dublin, in 1951, Dillon/Jivaka worked for a year in hospitals and clinics before deciding to join the Merchant Navy as a surgeon. Initially he intended to return to England after a year to pursue a position in brain research, but one year turned into six. During these years he traveled all around the world, returning to England in between months- or even years-long voyages. This turn in Dillon/Jivaka's life surely was influenced to some degree by an important episode that *Out of the Ordinary* does not discuss, namely his relationship with Roberta Cowell.

Cowell had contacted the author of *Self* in the late 1940s to seek advice for her own transition from male to female. Before long, as Hodgkinson and Kennedy have reported, Dillon was head over heels for Cowell, who apparently did not feel the same way. After several years of courtship and aid from Dillon (perhaps including some direct assistance with her medical transition), Cowell turned down his marriage proposal in 1951.³⁷ It is hard to imagine that this rejection, which took place just after his graduation from medical school, failed to influence his departure. Cowell's 1954 memoir recounts only their initial meeting without identifying him by name and without any indication of his feelings for her, but by then Dillon was out of the country.³⁸ Never again would he seek out a romantic relationship.

As Hodgkinson and Kennedy have pointed out, the relationship with Cowell opens up complicated questions about Dillon/Jivaka's views of gender and sexuality and about his broader relationship to social norms. While his earlier writing argues for compassion and outreach to those on the margins of gender and sexual norms, by the early 1950s he seems to have operated completely uncritically in what would now be termed a heteronormative framework. Reviewing correspondence from Dillon to Cowell, Hodgkinson has commented, "the letters reveal him by turns to be chauvinistic and importunate."[39] Indeed, Cowell reportedly did not appreciate his assumptions, expressed repeatedly in his letters, that she would take on the role of housewife once they married.[40] Patricia Leeson, a medical school friend to whom Dillon/Jivaka had confided his history, also described him as having "something of a reputation as a misogynist, and this is how he regarded himself, but it wasn't entirely accurate."[41] In *Out of the Ordinary* Dillon/Jivaka himself comments,

> With girls one had to be careful. No one seemed to suspect anything [about his history of transition] and I developed something of a reputation of being a woman-hater, since I made a point of treating them in a rather rough brotherly fashion, and sheered off if any showed any signs of being interested. One must not lead a girl on if one could not give her children. That was the basis of my ethics.[42]

Hodginson speculates that perhaps "he was protecting himself" with such bravado.[43] His earlier comments in *Out of the Ordinary* about refusing prior to transition to "take a woman and get over [his] repressions" arguably have a self-protective ring.[44] Statements like these, interspersed with moments of advocacy and social critique, add to the challenge of reading *Out of the Ordinary* and making sense of Dillon/Jivaka's life. It would be neither accurate nor fair to lay these biases at the foot of his transition, however, as if they were either an underlying cause or an inevitable byproduct of it. And so the question arises: was Dillon/Jivaka strongly for *or* strongly against the transformation of social norms? As Dr. Leeson might have put it, "not entirely."

This ambivalence is also visible in the stories of transnational encounter that Dillon/Jivaka records between 1952 and his 1958 exposure by the international press. On his first assignment, he describes reveling in the privileges of a white British officer. His initial reaction to "the most palatial [cabin] I ever would have," his personal Goanese servant, and crisp uniform was to stare at himself in the long mirror in disbelief, asking "could this really be me?"[45] From Singapore to Port Said, China to Calcutta, Dillon/Jivaka reveals aspects of the imperialist and ignorantly racist lens through which he viewed the world.[46] During one Christmas while in the Merchant Navy and docked in Japan, some Japanese waitresses come aboard, and

Dillon declares that their fascination with his beard is attributable to Japanese men's supposed inability to grow facial hair.[47] Descriptors such as "having breeding" crop up throughout the memoir as well, never bracketed with self-critique.[48] It was also during this period at sea that Dillon wrote to an official at Debrett's *Peerage*, where his brother Robert was listed as the only male heir to the baronetcy of Lismullen.[49] Could they please add him as the next in line?

At the same time, even as such scenes display an imperialism that Dillon/Jivaka never seemed able to shake, *Out of the Ordinary* also celebrates border crossings of class, race, and nation. In Durban, for instance, Dillon/Jivaka decries the presence of a "color bar" and lifts up the Mission to Seamen as one of the few places "where [segregation] could not be exerted, as a result of its constitution . . . and on filmshow night negroes, Indians, Chinese and Europeans, all seamen, sat together. May it long continue!"[50] In an early visit to India, prior to his exposure, he reflects on being overcharged by a rickshaw *wallah*, concluding that he was right to pay too much, since they were exploited.[51] On board ship, Dillon/Jivaka also habitually took up manual labor, such as carpentry and painting, work viewed by his fellow officers as considerably beneath his rank.

In addition to such physical practices, Dillon/Jivaka also actively sought to train his mind to loosen the grip of English aristocratic culture. The chapters covering this period of his life are replete with long quotations from the esoteric spiritual writers George Gurdjieff and Peter Ouspensky, circling around the theme of self-knowledge and the shedding of false "selves."[52] Interpersonal challenges with shipmates became the perfect, stress-inducing fodder for "the Work," for applying the principles of this thought system to his own life. During these years Dillon/Jivaka also read Tuesday Lopzang Rampa's *The Third Eye* and met up with the author in Ireland between voyages. Rampa's claims to have spent time in a Tibetan Buddhist monastery were publicly discredited just prior to Dillon/Jivaka's exposure. But Rampa had already inspired him to delve into Buddhist thought and to spend time in India practicing meditation after his next voyage.[53] A section of the *Suranagama Sutra* from Lin Yutang's *The Wisdom of China and India*[54] had further "struck [Dillon/Jivaka] as surpassing anything the West had yet produced on the problem of Perception; it was pure metaphysics."[55] All of these influences became fodder for intense introspection, a persistent desire for "spiritual evolution," and a determination to face "The Truth" in its most challenging forms. This determination would soon face its harshest test.

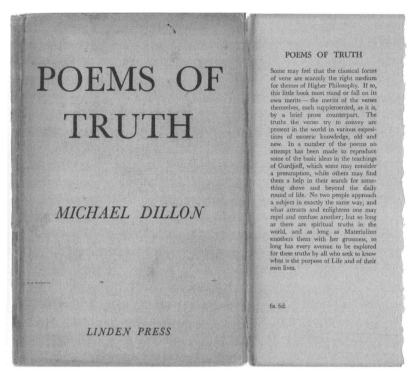

Book jacket of *Poems of Truth*, by Michael Dillon, 1957. This self-published collection of poems is strongly influenced by the esoteric spiritual philosophies of Pytor Demianovich Ouspensky and George Ivanovich Gurdieff.

Exposure

One morning in May 1958, as Dillon's ship, *The City of Bath*, sat docked in Baltimore, a steward handed him a cable that read, "Do you intend to claim the title since your change-over? Kindly cable *Daily Express*." Dillon/Jivaka reports: "at that moment my heart stood still. The secret that had been so well kept for fifteen years had at last leaked out, that I had been among the unfortunates who 'change their sex' and in addition was heir to a title."[56] Later, in a handwritten edit, he commented, "Here was the end of my emancipation!"[57] So significant was this moment to Dillon/Jivaka that he told it in his own Author's Introduction to *Out of the Ordinary*, thus using it to frame the entire memoir. A second telling of the episode, arising chronologically in Chapter 12, "The Last Voyage," describes in detail the reactions of shipmates and friends as well as Dillon/Jivaka's ten-day-

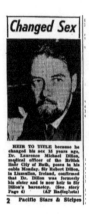

Changed Sex

HEIR TO TITLE because he changed his sex 15 years ago, Dr. Laurence Michael Dillon, medical officer of the British liner City of Bath, poses in his cabin Monday. Sir Robert Dillon, in Llanelian, Ireland, confirmed that Dr. Dillon was formerly his sister and is now heir to Sir Dillon's baronetcy. (See story Page 4)   (AP Radiophoto)
2   Pacific Stars & Stripes

"Changed Sex," *Pacific Stars and Stripes*, May 13, 1958. One of the many newspaper articles that linked Michael Dillon to his brother Robert's baronetcy title and revealed Dillon's gender history.

long exile to the starboard deck, away from the press's prying eyes. There, pacing back and forth, he hatched a plan to leave the ship upon its return to India. He would follow the advice of Lopzang Rampa, retreating to a monastery to meditate for two years before returning to England once the press had lost interest. By that summer the plan was in effect.

Into India

Two months prior to this trauma, in early March 1958, when the *City of Bath* stopped in Calcutta on its way to the United States, Dillon/Jivaka had visited the Mahabodhi Temple at Bodh Gaya, the site of the Gautama Buddha's enlightenment. There he had met Dhardoh Rimpoche, the man he would seek out after the public exposure. A guidebook picked up in a Calcutta bookstore had inspired him to set out for Bodh Gaya by rickshaw. Despite his ignorance of Indian dress, customs, and Buddhist rituals (including awkward attempts to greet lamas by shaking hands and shock at Dhardoh Rimpoche's "skirt-like" robes),[58] Dillon/Jivaka remarks, "The odd thing was that I felt perfectly at home here, a feeling quite inexplicable."[59] While pointedly stating that at the time, "I had no ideas about changing my religion whatsoever," a feeling of home drew him back.[60]

Once more in Calcutta on the eve of his departure from the Merchant Navy, Dillon/Jivaka turned to what would be the last chapter of his life with a decidedly Gurdjieffian framework. Transformation — or "reform" or "evolution" — of one's inner thoughts, the mind as opposed to the world, lies at the heart of this vision:

There is nothing for man in this world but conquest of his mind, of the way he takes the world in all its absurdities and pompous imaginings. What is it the Work teaches? "Remember the whole secret is, in this Teaching, not to try to change external circumstances, because if you do not change yourself and the way you take the repeating events of life, everything will recur in the same way. As long as you remain as you are in yourself you will attract the same problems, same difficulties, same situation but if you change yourself your life will change." And, "You cannot reform the world; you can only reform your way of taking the world."[61]

This vision points to the fundamental structure of *Out of the Ordinary*, whose two parts are divided into "Conquest of the Body" and "Conquest of the Mind." Another way of articulating Dillon/Jivaka's "work," in other words, is as a kind of self-mastery or conquest. And this term, conquest, helps render more apparent how Dillon/Jivaka's imperialist influences interfaced with and created challenges for his conversion to Buddhism.[62] Indeed, as this final chapter, entitled "Imji Getsul," unfolds against the larger historical backdrop of struggle between colonial Europe and postcolonial India, many of the rhetorical notions of conquest operating throughout the narrative now become literalized. At the same time, even while wrestling with this un-Buddhist conception of mastery, Dillon/Jivaka also expresses a Bodhisattva-like, altruistic desire to relieve the suffering of others. Indeed, the Author's Introduction to the memoir suggests from the very start that the narrative as a whole is meant to enlarge human understanding and in its own way to help halt the vicious cycles of rampant materialism, self-destruction, and oppression that Dillon/Jivaka saw all around him.[63]

The final chapter of *Out of the Ordinary* also introduces two white European figures that haunt the memoir's closing pages. The first is a French ex-Catholic nun, unnamed by both Dillon/Jivaka and his biographers, who "went back to France and wrote a book against Buddhism" after being ordained as a *getsulma* (female monastic novice) by Rimpoche. In addition to making accusations of sexual assault "against various Sikkimese and Bhutanese monks and Lamas as well as influential laymen," she was, Dillon/Jivaka asserts, "also being used by certain Communist agents to obtain information from these areas."[64] While only later would Jivaka meet this nun and hear of this incident, these events profoundly shaped his path to ordination. Because the local lamas were now extremely fearful of taking another European into the *sangha*, Rimpoche refused to meet Dillon. Instead, Rimpoche sent him to Urgyen Sangharakshita, a white English *bhikshu* with a mountaintop *vihara* in Kalimpong.

Upon meeting Sangharakshita, whom he only identifies as "the English bhikshu," Dillon divulged his entire history to this man, trusting him "as a fellow Englishman and a monk." Explaining the reason for his hasty departure from the Merchant Navy, he wanted to avoid further detection from a scandal-hungry press and begin his sojourn in the *sangha* with a clean slate. Sangharakshita reportedly reassured him, and as Dillon/Jivaka reports it, "anything I told him would be as if under the seal of the confessional, or as a medical confidence, and I trusted him because he was both a fellow Englishman and a monk. How misplaced that trust was I could not foresee."[65] Pagan Kennedy, who corresponded with Sangharakshita while researching *The First Man-Made Man*, has reported that he claims never to have offered that confidentiality.[66] Dillon/Jivaka, for his part, conveys this promise using the two most personal frameworks of confidentiality he valued: physician-patient privilege and the seal of the confessional. Less clearly stated but no less present is his faith in their shared national and ethnic identity. Upon this foundation of trust, Dillon accepted from Sangharakshita a new name, Jivaka, moniker of the Buddha's own physician.[67]

For four months, Jivaka paid five rupees a day to transcribe Sangharakshita's autobiography and memorize the recitations for the Pali puja, only to be repeatedly denied further readings in the dharma, the fundamental teachings of the Buddha. Not until Sangharakshita left for a three-month winter speaking tour could Jivaka immerse himself in the extensive library of the Maha Bodhi Society in Sarnath. There he read English translations of the Pali canon and received lower ordination as a *sramanera* or novice monk, renouncing his wealth and paying Sangharakshita the remaining £130 for his keep. But after three more months, Jivaka left Kalimpong, citing discomfort with Sangharakshita's paternalism toward the local Indian youths, whose unregulated noise throughout the monastery made conditions for meditation and writing impossible.[68] He also felt that Sangharakshita did not take Jivaka's monastic vocation seriously; when Jivaka inquired about higher ordination, the *bhikshu* essentially put him off.[69] Amid these challenging circumstances, Dillon/Jivaka still managed to publish *Practicing the Dhamapada* in 1959 and *Growing Up Into Buddhism* in 1960 and to begin work on *The Life of Milarepa*. With his move out of Kalimpong back to Sarnath, Jivaka began writing prolifically, publication being his only source of income. A number of these articles were published in the English Buddhist Journal *Middle Way*, the *Hindustan Times Sunday Weekly*, and the Maha Bodhi Society.[70]

During these months, as he increasingly aspired to higher monastic ordination, Jivaka intensively studied the Vinaya, the texts that govern

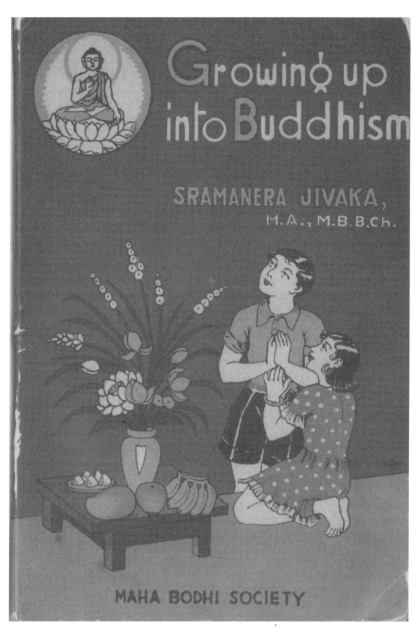

Book jacket of *Growing Up into Buddhism*, by Sramanera Jivaka, 1960. Framed through themes of self-mastery and the "search for truth," this primer on Buddhism was one of the first for English-speaking "Western" teenagers.

Buddhist monasticism. The fruit of that investigation was *A Critical Study of the Vinaya*, published by the Maha Bodhi Society in 1960, as well as a considerable amount of anxiety concerning his prospects, since one of those barred categories was a group labeled "third sex." Dillon/Jivaka explains:

> The first thing noticeable in reading the Buddhist canon is the casual reference not to two but to the three sexes, and there are many bans on various types of people from receiving the Higher Ordination among them being anyone belonging to this 'third sex.' Others are all those who have suffered any form of mutilation, loss of eye or nose or hand or foot, of being lame, etc., and with various diseases all bringing them under the ban. . . . But the keynote of Theravadin or Hinayana Buddhism is adherence to the letter of the law. The spirit is secondary. Whereas in Mahayana Buddhism it is the spirit that counts and the letter can be altered within the spirit. The spirit of the bans is to exclude undesirable people from the *sangha* or Monkhood. If a bodily defect is not accompanied by a mental or spiritual defect it is not regarded as requiring to be upheld as a ban.[71]

Ever since coming across Rampa's fantastical descriptions in *The Third Eye*, Jivaka had been drawn to Mahayana Buddhism. The Theravadin branch that Sangharakshita practiced and into which Jivaka had been ordained as a *sramanera* took a more rigid stance on the Vinaya prohibitions. But now, as Jivaka read Mahayana sources and talked with its practitioners, he decided to shift. As he continued his quest for higher ordination after his return from Rizong, he read the Vinaya with an emphasis on "the spirit of the bans," rather than "the letter," confident that someone like himself should not be prohibited.

Sangharakshita disagreed. When Jivaka sent him a note letting him know of his impending ordination, the English *bhikshu* immediately sent letters of protest, detailing Jivaka's history, and causing enough of a stir that the ceremony was put off.[72] An alternate path forward appeared when Jivaka was reordained as *getsul*, or novice monk in the Tibetan tradition, and invited to spend a season with the monks of Rizong Monastery in Ladakh, the story of which appears in *Imji Getsul*.[73] But even after this groundbreaking turn of events—for Jivaka was the first Westerner to be ordained a *getsul* and to be allowed into this remote monastery[74]—further stumbling blocks emerged.

First, a story appeared in the communist paper *The Blitz* that Jivaka was really a former Royal Naval Officer and British spy—in a sense the

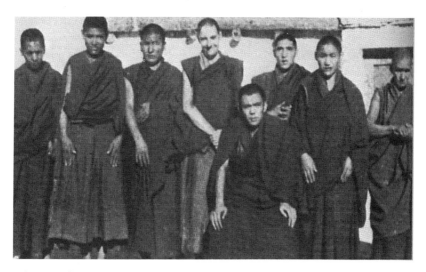

Lobzang Jivaka (*fourth from left, standing*) at Rizong Monastery in Ladakh, India, with some of the other *getsuls* and *gelongs*, including Kushok Shas (the head of Rizong Monastery, *seated*), 1960.

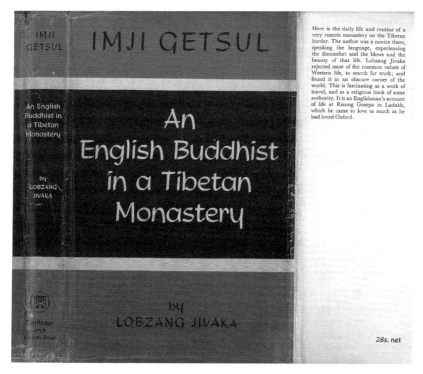

Here is the daily life and routine of a very remote monastery on the Tibetan border. The author was a novice there, speaking the language, experiencing the discomfort and the blows and the beauty of that life. Lobzang Jivaka rejected most of the common values of Western life, to search for truth; and found it in an obscure corner of the world. This is fascinating as a work of travel, and as a religious book of some authority. It is an Englishman's account of life at Rizong Gompa in Ladakh, which he came to love as much as he had loved Oxford.

28s. net

Book jacket of *Imji Getsul: An English Buddhist in a Tibetan Monastery*, by Lobzang Jivaka, 1962.

opposite of, or perhaps payback for, the French nun—merely posing as a monk in order to gain intelligence about Chinese activity in Ladakh. Never imagining anyone would believe such a story, he was shocked when President Nehru himself ended up defending him against this charge in the Lok Sabha, the lower house of the Indian Parliament. Nevertheless, as a result of this incident, his application to return to Ladakh was rejected, and he was turned back from the border. Then, to add further insult to injury, an article came out in a Hindi-language newspaper claiming that he was actually a former "lady-doctor" who had "changed her sex and had now become a Buddhist monk."[75] Furious about this latest outing, Dillon/ Jivaka was nevertheless amused at how this article might have embarrassed the authors of the previous one, accusing him of being a British spy, if "[anyone took] any notice what is in Hindi local rags."[76] Convinced that Sangharakshita's letters ultimately lay behind this last exposure, Dillon/ Jivaka wrote him requesting that he retrieve *Out of the Ordinary* from its trunk and send it to him.[77] To the twelve chapters that end with the eve of his arrival in India, he now added a compact account of the previous three years, plus an Author's Introduction dated May 1, 1962, his forty-seventh birthday.

The abrupt ending of *Out of the Ordinary* is characterized by an increasing disidentification with his history.[78] All his life, Dillon/Jivaka had been forced to confront the ways in which his body was read. Once more, as he contemplated "the end of [his] emancipation,"[79] the complexity of his body's ethnicity, nationality, class, and gender history had become undeniably interwoven with the colonial legacy of a newly independent India. Catalyzed by exposure, he finally sought to expose that complexity himself in all its unresolved ambiguity. With its dual-named authorship and temporal demarcation on his forty-seventh birthday, *Out of the Ordinary* was in a sense an exposure that was at the same time an attempted rebirth.

Conclusion: Sutures and Openings

Completed fifteen days prior to his death in Dalhousie, India, *Out of the Ordinary* is the last and most personally revealing of several published articles and books by Dillon/Jivaka. With the memoir, Dillon/Jivaka sought to suture the divide that he had consciously created between the various chapters of his life, filling in many of the gaps left by earlier publications.[80] Clearly, whether or not Dillon/Jivaka was aware that his life was coming to an end, he wanted to correct a lot of the misrepresentations of himself that he had felt were necessary in order to hide from earlier unwanted attention. But he also wrote *Out of the Ordinary* as an intervention into misrepresentations he felt were decidedly *un*necessary, namely those of the media, misrepresentations that haunted him enough to reverse his stance on talking about his transition. From the tone of the Author's Introduction, it is also clear that while Dillon/Jivaka did not enjoy telling the story of his "change over," he hoped that his writing might contribute to broader understanding and social acceptance for others with histories like his own.[81] Yet despite this sense of resolve, the narrative ends with a decided lack of resolution: the various strands of his life are not woven together with tidy completion.

And so ultimately, to read *Out of the Ordinary* is to open oneself to that lack of resolution as well as to the numerous complexities and nuances toward which we have sought to gesture in this introduction. In vocation and personhood, Dillon/Jivaka held numerous positions: author, doctor, auto mechanic, philosopher, athlete, *sramanera*, *getsul*, to name but a few. We readers are confronted by his extraordinary bravery in being the first and only man he knew with a trans-gender, -religious, and -national history. We are challenged to take note of the ways that Dillon/Jivaka expresses discomfort with class and gender passing while also failing to account for his upper-middle-class, white privilege to transition. And we are presented with an extraordinary series crossings—of gender, nation, class, and ethnicity, and of religion—even as Dillon/Jivaka accounts neither for his imperialist positionality to "export" Buddhism nor for his prevailing orientalist attitude toward his fellow novices at Rizong and Sarnath.

Ultimately, with great respect for the personhood of Michael Dillon/Lobzang Jivaka, we are gratified to open *Out of the Ordinary* to a wider readership, as he always intended. This publication may not have happened "in his own time," but we have striven to help it happen as much as possible "in his own way." We share Dillon/Jivaka's memoir with a sense of hope that its richness and complexity—its humanity—can now be assessed, critiqued, and appreciated for what it is.

NOTES

1. Liz Hodgkinson, *Michael née Laura: The Story of the World's First Female-to-Male Transsexual* (London: Columbus Books, 1989), 187.

2. Michael Dillon/Lobzang Jivaka, *Out of the Ordinary* (c. 1960–1962), Chapter 1.

3. "Doctor Chose a Tibetan Life. Heir to Baronetcy Died a Buddhist Monk," *Sunday Telegraph*, June 24, 1962. Cf. Hodgkinson, *Michael née Laura*, 189; Pagan Kennedy, *The First Man-Made Man: The Story of Two Sex Changes*,

One Love Affair, and a Twentieth-Century Medical Revolution (New York: Bloomsbury, 2007), 188.

4. The full name in which Dillon reregistered was Laurence Michael Dillon, and he went by Michael. To honor this hybrid authorial nomenclature, when we refer to the author in his narrator voice we will use the hyphenated "Dillon/Jivaka." When we refer to the historical person distinct from the text of the memoir, we will use the names Dillon or Jivaka, depending on context. We also use male pronouns to refer to all chapters of Dillon/Jivaka's life, including his female childhood and adolescent and college years, out of a sense that this convention most clearly respects his own articulation of his gender.

5. "She Switched Sexes," *Brief*, August 1954, 43; and "The Sex Change," *Man's Day* (c. 1953), cited by Joanne Meyerowitz, *How Sex Changed: A History of Transsexuality in the United States* (Cambridge, Mass.: Harvard University Press, 2002), 87–88, 306 n111. On Michael Harford, see "Woman Who Became Man to Come to Australia" in *The Advertiser*, December 16, 1953. Robert Allen, *But for the Grace* (London: W. H. Allen, 1954).

6. Michael Dillon, *Self: A Study in Ethics and Endocrinology* (London: William Heinemann Medical Books, 1946), 63.

7. Urgyen Sangharakshita (1925–) was ordained a *sramanera* in India, where he was the leader of a small community. He returned to England in 1967 and founded the Friends of the Western Buddhist Order and the Western Buddhist Order. In 2010 the group changed its name to the Triratna Buddhist Community. His writings are numerous, including *Precious Teachers: Indian Memoirs of an English Buddhist* (Birmingham: Windhorse, 2007), which has an entire chapter on Dillon/Jivaka entitled "The Secret Order of the Potala" (40–56); and *Moving Against the Stream: The Birth of a New Buddhist Movement* (Birmingham: Windhorse, 2004), in which he describes a dream of pulling Jivaka out of a deep pit (342–343).

8. Kennedy, *The First Man-Made Man*, 185–186. In *Precious Teachers* (55), which came out the same year as Kennedy's book, Sangharakshita reports having read *Out of the Ordinary*, of which there were apparently three original copies, and states that when Jivaka's book *Imji Getsul* arrived in the mail, he fully expected it instead to be *Out of the Ordinary*.

9. Hodgkinson, *Michael née Laura*, 187–188; Kennedy, *The First Man-Made Man*, 187.

10. Kennedy, *The First Man-Made Man*, 188.

11. As Dillon/Jivaka reports regarding the beginning of medical school where he would live very near his brother: "But what about Bobby? He lived but 26 miles from Dublin and would be very angry if his name was linked with mine since I was such a freak and had done the most outrageous thing in

changing over. He was desperately self-conscious about having me for a sister and he would never own me as a brother. And he did not." *Out of the Ordinary*, Chapter 5.

　　12. "Doctor Chose a Tibetan Life. Heir to Baronetcy Died a Buddhist Monk." *Sunday Telegraph*, June 24, 1962.

　　13. Joanne Meyerowitz *(How Sex Changed*, 87) notes that in the mid–twentieth century "the brief reports on female-to-males usually came from outside the United States, and compared with the frenzied reporting on male-to-females, their tone approached indifference."

　　14. Jamison Green, *Becoming a Visible Man* (Nashville, Tenn.: Vanderbilt University Press, 2004).

　　15. Kennedy, *The First Man-Made Man*, 188.

　　16. Hodgkinson, *Michael née Laura*; Kennedy, *The First Man-Made Man*.

　　17. Jay Prosser, *Second Skins: The Body Narratives of Transsexuality* (New York: Columbia University Press, 1998), 4, 101: "For transsexuality is always narrative work, a transformation of the body that requires the remolding of the life into a particular narrative shape." And, narrative functions as "a kind of second skin: the story the transsexual must weave around the body in order that this body may be 'read.'"

　　18. The term transgender, while used in the 1990s in critical distinction from "transsexual," became an umbrella term for those who transgress gender norms. It should be noted that Dillon/Jivaka himself never used "transsexual," let alone "transgender," to refer to himself despite the fact that the former term had come into usage by the time he wrote *Out of the Ordinary*. Furthermore, in *Self: A Study in Ethics in Endocrinology*, which he published in 1946, Dillon actively eschews the term "sex change," instead carving out conceptual space in and between the terms "homosexuality" and "intersex" (Dillon also uses the term "hermaphrodite," which is rejected in the contemporary intersex community, it is important to note). In *Out of the Ordinary* he uses language of change to refer to his transition (e.g., "changeover," "the change," or "effect a change") and of "intersex" to frame questions of causality (a brief reference in Chapter 5 aligns with several references in the 1958 newspaper articles disclosing his history of transition).

　　19. Dillon/Jivaka comments that his family's uncertainty as to how many days later she died reveals how little they knew her. *Out of the Ordinary*, Chapter 1.

　　20. Dillon/Jivaka, *Out of the Ordinary*, Chapter 3; Hodgkinson, *Michael née Laura*, 15, 24.

　　21. Dillon/Jivaka, *Out of the Ordinary*, Chapter 3.

　　22. Dillon/Jivaka, *Out of the Ordinary*, Chapter 5.

　　23. Dillon/Jivaka, *Out of the Ordinary*, Chapter 5.

24. Dillon/Jivaka, *Out of the Ordinary*, Chapter 5.

25. Dillon/Jivaka, *Out of the Ordinary*, Chapter 5.

26. Dillon/Jivaka, *Out of the Ordinary*, Chapter 5.

27. Dillon/Jivaka, *Out of the Ordinary*, Chapter 5.

28. Vern L. Bullough, *Science in the Bedroom: A History of Sex Research* (San Francisco: Basic Books, 1994), 129. Henry Rubin reports 1939 as the year in which testosterone was synthesized and explains that it took longer to appear on the market than estrogen. Indeed, endocrinologists had just discovered that testosterone was present in female bodies and that estrogen was similarly present in male bodies. Henry Rubin, *Self-Made Men: Identity and Embodiment Among Transsexual Men* (Nashville, Tenn.: Vanderbilt University Press, 2003), 41–42.

29. Dillon/Jivaka, *Out of the Ordinary*, Chapter 5.

30. Dillon/Jivaka, *Out of the Ordinary*, Chapter 5.

31. Dillon/Jivaka, *Out of the Ordinary*, Chapter 5.

32. As the memoir describes, the decision to apply to medical school was also significantly influenced by a "lady doctor," a friend of the Dillon family. Dillon/Jivaka, *Out of the Ordinary*, Chapter 5.

33. Harry Benjamin, *The Transsexual Phenomenon* (New York: Julian Press, 1966).

34. Dillon/Jivaka, *Out of the Ordinary*, Chapter 5.

35. Dillon/Jivaka, *Out of the Ordinary*, Chapter 5.

36. Harold Gillies and Ralph Millard, *The Principles and Art of Plastic Surgery* (London: Butterworth and Co., 1957). Cited in Kennedy, *The First Man-Made Man*, 79. Kennedy discusses this surgical intervention from pp. 59–113. In this, Kennedy expands upon previous discussions in Bernice Hausman, Jay Prosser, Joanne Meyerowitz, Henry Rubin, and Aaron Devor.

37. Hodgkinson, *Michael née Laura*, 85–97; Kennedy, *The First Man-Made Man*, 85–113.

38. Roberta Cowell, *Roberta Cowell's Story* (New York: British Book Center, 1954), 122–124.

39. Hodgkinson, *Michael née Laura*, 88.

40. Hodgkinson, *Michael née Laura*, 93.

41. Hodgkinson, *Michael née Laura*, 74.

42. Dillon/Jivaka, *Out of the Ordinary*, Chapter 6.

43. Hodgkinson, *Michael née Laura*, 74.

44. E.g., Dillon/Jivaka, *Out of the Ordinary*, Chapter 4.

45. Dillon/Jivaka, *Out of the Ordinary*, Chapter 8.

46. See, e.g., his description of Port Said: Dillon/Jivaka, *Out of the Ordinary*, Chapter 8.

47. Dillon/Jivaka, *Out of the Ordinary*, Chapter 9.

48. See, e.g., Dillon/Jivaka, *Out of the Ordinary*, Chapter 10.

49. He cites the entry as the only "remnant of my past surviving," suggesting the protection of his privacy as his motive, but then praises the official there for "acknowledg[ing] my claim to the baronetcy if I survived my brother." Dillon/Jivaka, *Out of the Ordinary*, Chapter 8. A change in Debrett's *Peerage* that was not picked up by Burke's *Peerage* ultimately led to the press inquiries that revealed Dillon's history.

50. Dillon/Jivaka, *Out of the Ordinary*, Chapter 10.

51. Dillon/Jivaka, *Out of the Ordinary*, Chapter 12.

52. See, e.g., Dillon/Jivaka, *Out of the Ordinary*, Chapters 10–12. The spiritual thought and practices of George Gurdjieff and Peter Ouspensky are known to have attracted a wide range of independent, creative, incisive people, a number of them women, including several lesbians, such as Jane Heap and Margaret Anderson (publishers of *The Little Review*) and the novelist Kathryn Hulme. Dillon/Jivaka briefly acknowledges that much of Gurdjieff and Ouspensky's thought is lifted from Buddhist dharma, or sayings of the Buddha.

53. Although still grateful for Lobsang Rampa's insight and advice, Dillon/Jivaka acknowledges Rampa's blatant cultural appropriation (particularly of Tibetan Buddhism) in the *Third Eye* and notes that if he had not been as ignorant of Buddhism when meeting Rampa he probably would not have associated with him. A white Irishman who never left the United Kingdom, Rampa was born Cyril Hoskin and claimed to channel the deceased Indian *gelong*'s spirit. Dillon/Jivaka, *Out of the Ordinary*, Chapter 11.

54. Lin Yutang, *The Wisdom of China and India* (New York: Random House, 1942).

55. Dillon/Jivaka, *Out of the Ordinary*, Chapter 12.

56. Dillon/Jivaka, *Out of the Ordinary*, i. Note that while the Foreword indicates this scene took place in March 1958, the articles that came out about Dillon were from May. It seems likely that the latter date is the correct one, since reporters would not have sat on this story for two months.

57. Dillon/Jivaka, *Out of the Ordinary*, Chapter 12.

58. Dillon/Jivaka, *Out of the Ordinary*, Chapter 12.

59. Dillon/Jivaka, *Out of the Ordinary*, Chapter 12.

60. Dillon/Jivaka, *Out of the Ordinary*, Chapter 12.

61. Dillon/Jivaka, *Out of the Ordinary*, Chapter 12.

62. Again it is striking that the self remains the center of Dillon's conquest at the end of *Out of the Ordinary* when he had written earlier on the dharma's central concept of Not-Self in *The Middle Way*.

63. Dillon/Jivaka, *Out of the Ordinary*, Author's Introduction.

64. Dillon/Jivaka, *Out of the Ordinary*, Chapter 13.

65. Dillon/Jivaka, *Out of the Ordinary*, Chapter 13.

66. Kennedy, *The First Man-Made Ma*n, 143–160, 171–190.

67. Jivaka, the name given to Dillon/Jivaka by Sangharakshita, was the name of the Buddha's physician. Sramanera is the title of a Theravadin male monastic novice after receiving lower ordination. Dillon/Jivaka also gave Sangharakshita his wrist watch and gold signet ring, which still causes some agony in the author as he remembers giving the family keepsake to the man who only caused more suffering.

68. Sangharakshita continued to feed the youths even when money ran out and the monks were starving. Dillon/Jivaka also makes the following vague comment regarding Sangharakshita and the youth. "The bhikshu, not at all averse to being left alone with his boys, agreed and set about raising the money for my fare and when he had it I departed." Dillon/Jivaka, *Out of the Ordinary*, Chapter 13.

69. Dillon/Jivaka, *Out of the Ordinary*, Chapter 13.

70. See Bibliography.

71. Dillon/Jivaka, *Out of the Ordinary*, Chapter 13.

72. Dillon/Jivaka, *Out of the Ordinary*, Chapter 13.

73. Lobzang Jivaka, *Imji Getsu*l (London: Routledge and Kegan Paul, 1962). So rare was such an experience, for a "Westerner," that his account of the experience remains in print today.

74. Dillon/Jivaka, *Out of the Ordinary*, Chapter 13.

75. Dillon/Jivaka, *Out of the Ordinary*, Chapter 13.

76. Dillon/Jivaka, *Out of the Ordinary*, Chapter 13.

77. Kennedy, *The First Man-Made Ma*n, 186.

78. We use the term "disidentification" to speak of Dillon/Jivaka's relation to his own history with an eye toward how José Estaban Muñoz uses the term in distinction from "identification" and "counteridentification." Muñoz describes the political repurposing of majoritarian culture by queers of color, and while Dillon/Jivaka is not a queer person of color, he is enacting a similar discursive move by writing his memoir to counter how the popular press was framing both his gender history and the gender histories of others at odds with their gender assignments at birth. José Estaban Muñoz, *Disidentifications: Queers of Color and the Performance of Politics* (Minneapolis: University of Minnesota Press, 1999), esp. 11–12.

79. Dillon/Jivaka, *Out of the Ordinary*, Chapter 12.

80. Hodgkinson, *Michael Née Laur*a, 188.

81. Notably, Dillon/Jivaka signs his introduction solely as Lobzang Jivaka, without his British name, invoking his religious authority as a *getsul* rather than tying it to his past Christian British identity. Coupled with Jivaka's insistence to give the readers of his memoir "a Right Sense

of Values," this frames the memoir through the ideology of the Bodhisattva vow, to lead others down the eightfold path to enlightenment and cause the cessation of suffering. Jivaka took the Bodhisattva vow in lieu of higher ordination and writes extensively about its mandates in *The Middle Way*. Dillon / Jivaka, *Out of the Ordinary*, 5, Chapter 13.

Out of the Ordinary

Understanding and Compassion

1

Deep black the night when the lightning flashed,
Which showed the foaming crests and spray flung high;
Sheer walls of water rearing to the sky
As waves on waves against each other crashed.
No rest, the struggle raging
As when a war is waging,
The sea against itself—against its will;
When suddenly a gentle Voice was heard,
Fraught with Compassion came the needful word:
"Peace!" Then the storm was stayed and all was still.

2

Tossed this way and that, a soul in torment,
Thoughts recurring o'er and o'er again,
Long wakeful nights and days of mental strain,
Love strove with hate and jealousy till spent.
No rest, the struggle raging
As when a war is waging,
A man against himself—against his will.
He took his life for lack of friendly hand,
For want of one to say: "I understand."
This time no peace was there, though all was still.

—Michael Dillon

Author's Introduction

If men and women had a Right Sense of Values there would never have been any need for this book to have been written and published—but then if the world had a Right Sense of Values it would not be in the mess it is today.

One day in March of 1958 when I was serving as surgeon on board the cargo-passenger ship, *City of Bath*, and we were lying in Baltimore, loading for India, I went down to my surgery as usual before breakfast to attend to any of the crew who might be sick. A steward put his head in and gave me a cable. It read: "Do you intend to claim the title since your change-over? Kindly cable *Daily Express*."

At that moment my heart stood still. The secret that had been so well kept for *fifteen* years had at last leaked out, that I had been among the unfortunates who "change their sex" [he adds by hand: "and in addition was heir to a title"]. Before I had recovered from the shock the company agent came in and told me there were two reporters from the *Baltimore Sun* waiting in his office on the wharf and they wanted to see me. Putting the cable in the waste-paper basket and lighting my pipe to steady myself, I fetched my cap and went ashore. There was nothing that could be done to stave off the inevitable.

The rest of the story can be read in these pages. But by what sense of values did a newspaper editor and reporter think that five minutes' light reading by the public justified such an assault on a doctor's career? Or did they stop to think at all? When they realized the secret was an old one, might they not have considered that publicity was unsought and, having found I was a doctor, although they did not know at first where practicing, might they not have gauged that destructive impact on his job such an unnecessary denouncement would be? And finally, when they had discovered I was in the Merchant Navy, surely some feeling of what life on a ship would be like under such circumstances might have been expected from them in virtue of their calling themselves human?

My career at sea would have been ended anyhow by this thoughtless act. The fact that circumstances quite apart from these were leading me on to a new life in any case, of which they knew nothing, makes no difference to the inhumanity of the deed. But, in fact, for many years the Search for Truth had also dogged me and release from the ship led me to take it up more thoroughly than heretofore and a little before I had intended to leave the sea to do so.

Was it small wonder that these joint effects eventually became the cause of my renouncing the world with its mistaken set of values, and becoming a monk? At the time of writing this nineteen years have passed since I was reregistered with the State and all my former troubles were ended by the good offices of one enlightened man with the courage of his convictions and the skill to carry them out. The conquest of the Body proved relatively easy. But the conquest of the Mind is a never ending struggle and it still goes on. Yet it is the sole purpose of our life on Earth. Not the pursuit of happiness or pleasure, not to leave our offspring socially better off than we were, nor yet to amass money or power nor take our evil to other planets [added by hand: "under the guise of Progress"]. But to evolve spiritually, no more, no less.

All must run in the race of Life but not all start from scratch. Some are heavily handicapped, some lightly, some are forward of the starting line at birth. But all must still run as best they can. One handicapped runner plods along, slowly catching up a little on the rest and then another runner sees him and, for the sake of applause, trips him up. He falls flat on his face in the mud and the others pass him by with grins and jeers, although here and there a sympathetic glance is thrown. He picks himself up, scrapes the mud off his face so that he can see where he is going and again starts off determinedly, and once more he slowly gains ground. As he joins the main body of runners another cuts across and quite deliberately sends him flying again, for fear he may pull ahead. Will he lie there, this time, and give up the unequal struggle? No! For the third time he rises and begins to run. By now more of the competitors realize what is going on and public opinion is [crossed out: "turning against the saboteurs"; added: "swinging"]. The Goal lies ahead. He will either reach it or die in the attempt, but he will never give in.

This book is the expression of that determination, and in its attempt to give a better understanding to people it has a message, for with understanding comes an improved sense of values, and Right Viewpoint is the first step on the Path to emancipation from the fetters of materialism and all that is driving man insanely to his own destruction.

Lobzang Jivaka
Sarnath, May 1, 1962

Conquest of the Body

Birth and Origins

I was born on May 1, 1915, in a nursing home in Ladbroke Grove in the borough of Kensington. The nursing home is no longer in existence but one can still read "Ladbroke Grove" on the front of some of the London buses. Although never having gone with one to its destination, I have often had the urge to see the area whereon my eyes first rested, changed though undoubtedly it must be by now. I had been preceded fifteen months before by a brother who had been a seven months baby. He had caused his mother much trouble in labor and in anxiety for some time afterwards, since he was naturally delicate. Then, all too soon, I followed and after six or perhaps ten days she died, of puerperal sepsis it seems.

The vagueness of information on the whole matter is due to the fact that none of my family knew her. For some reason our father, who had not married until the age of forty-seven, never took his wife down to Folkestone where his aged parents were still alive and four of his sisters resident. Only one sister who happened to be staying at the time in London, and a niece of his, attended the wedding. The sister, our Aunt Evie to-be, said that our mother was a fine looking woman, big and handsome, and our cousin, Auntie Daphne, said that she was much addicted to playing bridge while carrying me and she had often wondered whether the baby would be a bridge player. Long before I ever knew of this I had expressed an intense dislike of bridge and would never learn to play it, thus saving myself much time and money in future days while I was at sea.

A further source of information was to come many, many years later from my mother's only surviving sister in Sydney, Australia, when I was a Merchant Navy Surgeon. But that must wait until it occurs in its chronological order. It was she who maintained that my mother lived for ten days and not six and that she died suddenly when almost on the point of leaving the nursing home.

Be that as it may, on our father's side we are Anglo-Irish and on our mother's side Australio-German. I always regretted the German, but what could one do about it? It seems that our maternal grandfather emigrated from Germany to Australia with his wife and family, but his wife, far from being German, too, was an Irish girl from Cork, so that the Irish blood runs the more thickly in our veins. He, too, had a large family, but of them all our mother alone showed signs of independence of spirit, abjuring the Catholic faith in which she had been brought up (as, indeed in time did several of her brothers and sisters), and determined to see what lay beyond the confines of Sydney Harbor.

Just under what circumstances a young lady in the first decade of this century could have managed to break away and go a-sailing off alone, has not been discovered, but it seems that she landed first in South Africa and there married a man named MacLiver who owned a ranch or a fruit farm or the like and was very happy with him. Then one day disaster overtook them. Her husband was entertaining a friend to lunch and wished to show off the fine points of a new pony he had acquired, for he was an enthusiastic horseman. The horse put its foot into a rabbit hole and threw its rider and to the horror of the wife and the guest watching from the verandah, rolled on its master, disemboweling him. At the time our mother-to-be was with child and the shock caused a miscarriage and long illness. It was after she had recovered from this that she left South Africa and came to England where she met our father in a boarding-house and it appears it was a case of love at first sight. Whether it was because she was technically a Roman Catholic whereas his family was rigidly Protestant, that prompted his not bringing her to meet his parents, I do not know. At any rate no better explanation has been offered.

Hence it was that, although other children were accustomed to having two families, in the shape of aunts and uncles, multiple grandparents and cousins, to us there was only one family and that was the Dillons. True, as children, we had an occasional letter to write to an aunt in Australia, the place which had swans on its stamps, but there was no connection in our minds between her and the other aunts who surrounded us from morning till night. And how that came about was as follows:

Our father, it appears, was somewhat of a weak character and had already ruined a promising career in the Royal Navy by drink which habit he was to keep through life, although possibly for the one year of a happy marriage, he may have abjured it. As it was he was completely demoralized by his wife's sudden and unexpected death and he blamed it on to me. He refused to so much as see me, but arranged with his favorite sister, who lived with her parents in Folkestone, to come to London and fetch the two babies and bring them up in the tall, six-storey house in Westbourne Gardens and he would contribute weekly to their upkeep. Employ a nanny and give them all they needed but keep them away from him, especially that new one! And so we came to Folkestone.

The atmosphere was Victorian, or at the best Edwardian, since two generations separated the new arrivals from the youngest of the resident aunts and at least four from our grandparents. Our grandfather was a fine character by all accounts and I lived with him for one year before he died at the age of ninety-six. I have ever since wished that I had been old enough to talk with him for his experience of the changing world must have been fascinating.

He was born in 1820 and followed the army as did many of his forebears. He lived in the days when commissions were bought and not earned and my brother still has the letters patent signed by Queen Victoria giving him his different ranks. He became a major in the Crimean War and after that decided it was time to retire and settle down to raise a family. So with the rank of Lieutenant Colonel he took to himself a young lady from Malta where he was, I believe, for a while Governor, whose name was Mills and who is the person remembered as "Granny." By her he had seven children, all but one of them girls, which accounts for the bevy of aunts that were to be ever present.

After Malta they had all gone to live in Brussels where the older girls were educated, learning it seemed little more than French, but our father was sent to school at Westward Ho! in Devon and was a schoolfellow of Rudyard Kipling.* When they were in their teens they came to Folkestone

---

* Westward Ho! is a seaside village established a decade after the 1855 publication of Charles Kingsley's popular book of the same title.

and Toto became the belle of the ball held at Shorncliffe Garrison* and, indeed, photographs show her as immensely attractive in her youth; but she was too "nervous" to marry, although she had an album of pictures of her admirers. Only three of them did marry. One, the eldest, Auntie Grace, lived in Worthing, because she had suffered from asthma since the age of two and Folkestone air did not suit it. Her husband had died before we were born. The second eldest, Auntie Kate, also married, but her husband, too, had died before we came, although her two daughters were given the courtesy title of Auntie, since they were grown up. But her two sons lived elsewhere and played no part in our lives. It was one of these daughters who had been present at our father's wedding.

The third eldest was the favorite of our father, one year younger than he, and she was the one who was to have the main shaping of our earliest years. She had been born on the island of Malta when Grandfather was living there, and so had been christened Melita, the old Roman name for the island, but she had always been called Tottie, a common nickname for girls of that period. In our early efforts to talk we had somehow converted this to Toto and henceforth the new name stuck. Next to her came Daisy, four years younger than Toto and four years older than the twins who were born sixteen years after the eldest child. They were identical, one right-handed, the other left, and no one outside the family could ever tell them apart. Time and again one would be accosted as an acquaintance by a stranger and would have to embarrass him or her by denying any acquaintanceship.

They were called Maudie and Evie, or Evelyn, and they were quite famous at Wimbledon in the days when tennis of a public nature was considered to be rather forward for young ladies. Mavrogadato was their contemporary, a name I often heard in my childhood, and Suzanne Lenglen was hardly beginning when the partnership, which covered the court with one right-handed racquet and the other left-handed, broke up through Evie marrying. Her husband was an Engineer in the Indian Civil Service and she departed with him to India where, in Calcutta, her daughter Joan was born. In time, Joan was to become as a sister. Before Aunt Evie's son was born, however, her husband, our Uncle Joe, died of pneumonia and she returned to England with one baby and carrying a second, a boy, Leslie,

---

* Shorncliffe Garrison refers to an army training camp in Folkestone, England. First established in the late eighteenth century during the Napoleonic Wars, it became an important military staging post for both World War I and World War II.

who therefore never knew his father. Thus with six aunts and no uncles we lived in an all-feminine atmosphere.

We had some cousins who were famous in Toronto, Ontario, as leading members of the United Empire Loyalists, a name scarcely heard these days, but that of General Henry Brock is still remembered there. His wife took up the family tree as a hobby and composed what she termed *The Generation Book*, with information culled from many sources which seem to have been authentic enough. So, as we grew older we learned that we were descended from an ancient King of Ireland, O'Niall King of Tara, who lived in 595 A.D.—a long enough time ago. His son Logan Dilune killed the son of another Prince and fled to France to escape his father's wrath. What happened in between I do not recall but a descendent of his, Sir Henry Delion, went to Ireland from France in the train of John of Gaunt and was granted large estates in the county of Roscommon which was at one time known as Dillon country, as his name became. My brother could resuscitate the title of Earl of Roscommon if he wished but having no issue it is not worth the trouble and expense.

The next in line to have bearing on our lives was Sir John Talbot Dillon, first baronet of the present baronetcy, an eighteenth century scholar and traveler who, although a staunch Protestant, worked for the representation of Catholics in Parliament and received the title of Baron of the Holy Roman Empire for himself and his heirs in perpetuity from the Emperor of Austria. We do not use foreign titles in England but the French branch of our family uses it. In any case by a decree of King George V, the "in perpetuity" ceases since foreign titles are no longer to be handed down although present holders may retain them. Thus was my brother informed when the Act was passed.

The picture of Sir John Talbot appeared in a copy of the *Gentlemen's Magazine*, date unknown, for our Aunt Evie, who was an amateur artist as well as tennis player, reproduced a black and white sketch of it which used to hang in my room before I gave up my house and property.

From him stemmed the French branch of the family, the Dillon-Cornecks, who are therefore distant cousins. One member I have met and enjoyed the hospitality of his house whenever my ship docked in Singapore, since he was a banker out there until he retired. And to a generation or two ago the name of the Dillon Regiment in France would also have been well known. But modern warfare has made a volunteer Irish regiment out of date and it was disbanded but recently. One of its Colonels, Timothy Dillon, was guillotined in the French Revolution.

The Dillon-Cornecks came from the youngest daughter of Sir John whose choice of a husband did not accord with that of her father and the couple eloped to France and settled there. His eldest son, however, began the line of which Viscount Dillon is the representative.*

If the modern reader finds so much about the aristocracy tiring, let him bear in mind that this was the background that was rammed into us from infancy, and which has produced in me the ultra-Englishman personality which has hampered me so much in recent years and to which reference was made in my book *Imji Getsul* as being one of the chief reasons for the need to go to a Tibetan monastery in Ladakh to try and break some of it down. I was brought up to believe in the superiority of the Englishman, and of Englishmen, of the superiority of the aristocracy of which, apparently, the Dillons formed no small part. What the English aristocracy did was "done," what it did not do was "not done," and this was as irrevocable as the laws of the Medes and Persians! And the effect of this upbringing is still apparent and in no wise can I shake it off despite that I have myself done at last what the English aristocracy just don't do in becoming a Buddhist monk in the Tibetan Order—unheard of before.

Apart from this one scholar and from the poet Thomas Wentworth Dillon of the Roscommon branch, there were none who were academically minded in the family until my own advent. Soldiering was the favorite occupation and Colonels abound in our annals. Our father, however, either chose, or had chosen for him, the Royal Navy as a career. For this there had been but a single precedent: an illegitimate son of Sir John Talbot had become a naval officer and risen to the rank of Commander in Chief of the Red. Doubtless naval types will understand the significance of that; it is beyond me who sullied the family record by joining the Merchant Navy, which I was told most definitely by Toto was not for *gentlemen!*

He became a midshipman on the *Britannia*, a famous training ship and his companion midshipmen were the future King George V, the Duke of Clarence and Duke of York. Only one story is told of this. Catapults were favorite playthings with the middies, and equally anathema to the officers and so were banned on pain of beating. One day, someone having been hit by a catapult, all the midshipmen had to line up to empty their pockets in front of their naval schoolmaster. The offender was the Duke of Clarence who rather meanly slipped the catapult into the pocket of my father without his realizing it. But standing on the other side of him was the Prince of

---

* To this sentence Dillon/Jivaka added a bracketed note: "needs checking if the Dillon Reg belonged to the Viscounts' line! I believe it did."

Wales, George V to-be, who did see, and he reached round the back of my father, pulled out the catapult and threw it overboard, while the officer was engaged in searching further up the line.

Our father rose to rank of Lieutenant and then, unfortunately, having discovered the delights of alcohol, he narrowly escaped being cashiered, it being only the influence my grandfather had in the Mediterranean at that time, apparently, which enabled him to be withdrawn quietly and sent home. It was a pity when he had had the best of good starts.

What he did after that I do not know. In a way he had something of the artistic temperament, for he could draw and paint quite well and play the piano and he even composed a waltz which he entitled *Mione* or "My One." He wrote one novel, too, *The Prince's Predicament*, which was Puritanical and a typical product of the era. He paid to have it published and distributed it among his friends. In my teens I acquired it and found it readable but no masterpiece.

Of the aunts, as has been said before, Toto took precedence. All her life she had succeeded in having her own way and in being coddled by the simple expedient of pretending to be delicate and to have "nerves," that convenient complaint of the young Victorian Miss. She was indulged by her father without whom she would never travel anywhere since she said she was afraid to go alone. This was a major point of my own upbringing, for she wished to make me as she herself was, and from earliest times she tried to mollycoddle me and would not let me out of her sight or go anywhere without her; and as she could scarcely be persuaded to go anywhere herself, I saw only a little outside Folkestone until nearly grown-up.

On the other hand the house was admirably suited for children for it was one of a square built around public gardens, which comprised a large center of grass which would take six tennis courts, a gravel path around and then, the joy of joys, "the bushes." It was in the bushes that we played with the other children, subject to a certain reservation, climbing trees as we grew old enough, swinging on the huge, or apparently huge, garden gate, having a "shop" on its top bar and the like.

The house itself had no private garden, bar a tiny backyard where a solitary hydrangea grew, and a basement area in front, like all the houses of that period, since it had about seven steps up to the front door. On the top step our grandmother would sit, unable to walk since she had had a stroke and the only way we remembered her was the one side of her face pulled down from paralysis, and the red conjunctiva of her left eye exposed, which still remains vividly in my memory. When she went out it was in a bath chair, pushed by our aunt Daisy, who devoted her whole life to looking after her mother and later, to looking after Toto, as she conceived of it, and regrettably never married, for really she was of a sweet nature, if she had not had so misguided a sense of duty, and the life she led must have become almost intolerable. She was permanently afflicted with what she always described as her "hayfever," although in fact I was later to discover she had a slow-growing nasal polypus, which all but blocked the cavity and was the cause of much of her trouble. At the time of writing this she is still alive, in her 92nd year, the last of the sisters. She was the "intellectual" one of the family, reading widely in literature including the classics in translation and she, too, was musical, but not so much so as Toto, who had an excellent ear although she never learned to read music. The twin aunts and myself, on the other hand, suffered from the same defect, neither ear nor voice, although my brother followed the other tendency and played the piano well.

This then was the background into which I was thrust at the age of six weeks, to be reared on Glaxo given by a Nanny, or what was to become a succession of Nannies of the old fashioned type, and in a nursery, in the old fashioned way. Shortly after my arrival in Folkestone it was thought fit that I should be christened, since that matter had escaped the attention of my distraught father, and as there was no opposition from anyone I was named after my mother, Laura Maude, and this I remained to my intense disgust, until 1943 when I was enabled to re-register and became Laurence Michael.

CHAPTER 2

The Nursery

After you had climbed laboriously up those seven wide steps to the front door and passed Granny sitting in her chair on the top step in the right hand corner, you went through one door and were then confronted by another, with a bilious shiny yellow varnish on it and starred glass, so that you could not see through it into the hall, in which there was a tall stand for coats, hats and umbrellas and with a silver tray for visiting cards. On the left was the dining room and beyond it again the sitting-room, and at the end of the passage a tiny room known as the Piggery, where it seems Maudie and Evie, as children, were allowed to play, away from their elder sisters.

The dining room had a huge table in the middle with leather backed chairs all around and there was a long cane sofa across one corner. But the fascinating thing was the lift. When we came to the stage of having breakfast and lunch with the grownups there would be an ominous rumble from the depths which grew louder and then the maid would open the doors of the lift and out would come the meal from its shelves. Then the dirty dishes would be put back in and the maid would pull the cords and with another rumble all would disappear again into the depths below. Often I wished

I could raise the courage to climb in and go down too, but the darkness rather frightened me and I would start to put my knee on the ledge and hop out again quickly before Bobby could pull the cords.

However, on coming in from our morning walk we would have to go straight upstairs first and the stairs had a magnificent broad mahogany rail, down which, in due course we would slide again, for there was a flat whorl at the bottom and no knob to hit yourself on, and sliding down the banisters was a never-ending source of delight when we grew old enough for it.

At the top of the first flight there was a little room round a corner where every morning we were expected to go to "do our business." It was the old-fashioned type with a step up to the throne and a pan with blue flowers stamped on the white porcelain, and it had a handle which you pulled up instead of the later-devised flush which you pulled down.

Climbing those stairs was quite an effort for they seemed very steep and there were many of them. I can still remember the first time I made a determined effort to put each foot on a successive step, and succeeded. "Look, Nannie, I can walk like a grown-up," I cried in satisfaction. "Yes, yes, dear," she said casually, not realizing what a tremendous feat I had performed.

If you did not wish to go round the corner you still had a few more stairs before you reached the landing on which were both the nursery and the drawing room. Of the former, oddly enough, I can recall no more than the two cots each side of Nannie's bed, but the drawing room had a huge glass mirror along one wall in front of which we would, in time, have to practice steps when we began dancing lessons. There were sundry armchairs and a green carpet and a sofa. But this room was only used for parties when there were special visitors, and then we would be carefully dressed up and brought down at tea time to be shown off and be given an iced cake or sweet biscuit. Fortunately, we never had to recite at these functions like some of our young friends. Less special visitors were entertained in the sitting room, whither, in any case, we were allowed to come down at five o'clock every evening to play for an hour and to have a sweet before we went to bed at six o'clock. None of these modern late hours for pseudo-Edwardian children!

It was at one such tea party in the sitting room that I had just climbed up into an armchair when I was violently sick over the arm. Hauled off back to the nursery I was rated for not having said I felt sick so that I should not have come down. In vain I protested that I had not felt in the least sick till that moment. No one believed me. Later when a medical student I read somewhere about sudden spontaneous vomiting as being a normal feature of childhood, and felt vindicated.

Above the nursery was Toto's room. Daisy's and Maudie's I do not remember at all, but on the top story, very high up, the cook general and the two maids slept in attics with sloping ceilings, for in those days there was no lack of home help. Also somewhere up there Daisy had her photographic "dark room" for she was a keen amateur photographer and won many prizes and cups for her pictures.

As will have been gathered, we had the old-fashioned Nanny, or rather a series of them, to attend upon us. Perhaps my earliest recollection of all is of sitting in a high chair having bread and milk from the then Nanny and of Toto coming into the room, seizing the bowl and shouting at her. I learned later that one Nanny was excessively dirty and let me come out in sores so that I had to be bathed all over in boracic lotion, so perhaps it was this one and my bowl had not been clean.

But the only early Nanny who remains in my memory was Swaffer, by which surname she was always called by Toto in keeping with the custom of the era. Swaffer was apparently very tall, thin and angular and she wore a long grey dress that did right up to the throat with buttons and with an apron on top of it. She was very staid and strait laced, or so it seemed to us. It was because of this aspect of her that I can remember Armistice Day of the Great War.* We were standing in the middle of the nursery floor watching Nanny dry the dishes after some meal. Then the door opened and someone put her head in and said something. Immediately Nanny threw the dishcloth up to the ceiling caught it again and rushed out of the room, while we stood openmouthed at such surprisingly abandoned behavior. Then we were told to hang out our little Union Jacks. The War had ended!

The War had naturally been a part of our lives, at least in so far as "soldiers and sailors" had figured in the prayer which we said every morning and evening, "soldiers-and-sailors-to-make-us-good-children-to-mark-us-with-grace-for-Jesus-Christ's-sake-amen," and also in virtue of the fact that they were to be seen everywhere about the town. Before Armistice Day there is another recollection. Bobby and I were standing with Swaffer on top of that steep hill that goes down to Folkestone Harbor, later to be renamed the Road of Remembrance, because so many soldiers went

---

* On the day that came to be called Armistice Day—November 11, 1918—the allies of World War I signed an agreement with Germany to end the war.

down it who never returned to climb up it again on to the Leas. On this day a company of soldiers was marching down the hill, singing and laughing on their way and we waved out little flags at them. One Tommy turned and grinned broadly at us and it is this that I remember.

But it was a soldier who led to the downfall of Nanny Swaffer—the legless soldier. He had lost both legs below the knees and had a chair which went when he turned a handle. But Nanny began going steady with him it seems, as the phrase goes, and took to pushing his chair with one hand and my pram with the other, while Bobby toddled along behind. One day we reached the Burlington Hotel which had been taken over as a military hospital. He got out of his chair by simply falling forward and then proceeded to climb up the steps of the hotel on the stumps of his knees. I watched him with complete detachment. But the aunts apparently took exception to Nanny's combined operations and she was summarily sacked, for we might pick up all sorts of bad language from a mere Tommy. Doubtless had she kept her attentions to her afternoons off no one would have minded.

The double pram which we had at first and out of which, it was said, Bobby threw me, the first time I took my seat in it opposite him, soon gave place to a go-cart and it was from the go-cart that I first made the acquaintance of a young gentleman who went out for airings while still sharing a double pram with his elder brother. No one knew then that his face would become well known to the cinema world, or that the name of David Tomlinson would be synonymous with comic films. But David Tomlinson was a near contemporary of mine, and after the pram stage we met at children's parties although we were never close friends.

While still in the go-cart stage there occurred the first sign of what the future was to have in store. One morning we were being dressed to go to the barber when I inadvisedly said: "I want my hair cut like Bobby's." Nanny only laughed and said: "Don't be silly, you can't, you're a little girl and he's a little boy." When we were at the hairdressers, some devil prompted her to say: "Tell the barber what you said in the nursery." Embarrassed, I tried to pretend I had forgotten, but she persisted so at last I came out with it defiantly: "I want my hair cut like Bobby's." They both laughed uproariously, as I knew they would, and it remained as a bob with either a slide or a ribbon. Bobby, on the other hand, suddenly one day demanded that his hair should be tied up with a ribbon since I had one, and he cried until one was put on him, but he only wore it for that one afternoon.

In those days we used to bathe together and although I was naturally aware of a difference between us it never registered specifically with me. We loved the bath and there was a prolonged struggle to get us out, until either Nanny or Toto hit upon the bright idea of telling us we would go down the plughole with the water if we stayed in after the plug was pulled out. Thereafter, as soon as a hand was put on the chain we scrambled out squealing in fear.

Visitors who had found favor in our eyes, also were asked to come and see us in our bath. Why this so appeals to children I do not know, but I have myself been asked by children many times and in that classic of the nursery, *Winnie the Pooh*, Christopher Robin makes the same request to an approved grown-up. But Winnie the Pooh was a little after our time.

One evening, Toto came into the bathroom and said "Get out quickly, your Daddy has come." Daddy! Once before he had come, curiosity apparently having got the better of him, but I did not remember his visit, and this time I have only a faint recollection of a dark-suited figure who came to see us in bed in the nursery. No more than that.

With the departure of Swaffer we acquired a nursery-governess, since Bobby must have been five and myself four by then and it was time that we began to learn. We had copy books with pothooks, but of learning to read I remember nothing, and have been told that I surprised everyone one day by reading something aloud at the age of five. No one knew that I could.

Toto now used to take us out shopping with her sometimes and on one such occasion, right in the middle of the town, in Guildhall Street, alongside the Town Hall, my little knickers fell down. No one noticed that I was getting left behind as my feet became entangled with my nether garments until Bobby looked round and piped shrilly: "Baby's knickers have come down." So I stood quite unperturbed in a pool of lace and cambric while they were pulled up again and then trotted on, leaving it to my aunt to be embarrassed.

On Sundays we went to the Children's Service in the afternoon, for the family were all devoutly Protestant and religious education began early. Not for us the Sunday School, however, for that was for the children of the tradesmen, and would never do! That was held at two o'clock and after it they all trooped into church for the children's service too, sitting on the left aisle while we, the elite, all sat on the right. The Vicar was the now famous W. H. Elliott, who had a passion for children and a way with them, though he was less popular with the grownups. He had a rooted objection to visiting or general parish work and would never call unless sent for in case of illness or death. On the other hand, he could never spend enough time with the children and every winter he organized a children's play, for he was a born actor himself. Thus did we achieve a stage career at an early age. And although not socially minded, the Vicar had packed churches for every sermon, for he could preach brilliantly and later became famous for his radio broadcasts.

For Sundays and parties we had sailor suits, in keeping with the patriotic fashions for children of that post war time. For best were white jumpers with large blue collars, quite authentic, and cuffs to match, a black silk tie with a lanyard wound about it but no whistle on the end. After much badgering I managed to procure a whistle for mine, but it lasted only one day for my persistent blowing of it was too much for the aunt's nerves which had always been so bad. Bobby had duck trousers and I a white kilt, and for everyday wear a blue kilt and he blue shorts. But he also had a pilot coat with brass buttons and anchors on them and this I envied so much that, having already learned the value of sustained effort, I finally managed to acquire one, too. It was a *manly* coat, so my child mind thought, and I loved it. We had pillbox sailor hats, too, Bobby's with H.M.S. *Revenge* on it and mine with H.M.S. *Renown*.

At some time during these early years Bobby broke his leg after having already been in bed for a period with what was termed "rheumatism" in his knees. Or did the rheumatism come after? I am not sure. It was one evening when we were playing in the big public garden, having been left alone for a short while since all seemed safe, that we started jumping over a tennis net that had been wound nearly down. Bobby caught his foot in the net and fell, one leg cocked up in the air. The nurse of some other child ran across to him and he maintained ever after that it was her efforts to disentangle his foot from the net that broke his leg.

He was carried back to the house and the doctor came and the same evening he was taken to the Bevan Nursing Home in Sandgate, where I later went to visit him to find him surrounded by toys and sweets and with his leg hung up on a kind of beam. When he came out he had to wear an iron since plaster-of-Paris had not been invented in those days and there was no physiotherapy, and so he went into long blue sailor's trousers to hide it.

Quite early on we learned some lessons in finance. We began with threepence a week pocket money of which one week we had to put one penny and the next twopence into our saving boxes, a tin sailor for Bobby and a red coated-busbied soldier for me. The pennies went in through the tops of their headgear. This did not leave very much for the necessities of childhood, such as tin soldiers, paints or the like. But there were other sources of income, as well as birthdays. One of these was an old gentleman called Mr. Fort. He had been a friend of our grandfather and he never met us but he gave us each a penny.

One day we were sitting with the current nursery-governess on a seat in Radnor Park when we saw him coming and we hugged ourselves in delight at the thought of the penny. But he only said a few words and passed on. Dismayed we looked at each other, "He's forgotten our pennies," one said to the other. "Shall we remind him?" And two little voices piped up: "Mr. Fort, you've forgotten our pennies!" He turned back concerned and said he was very sorry he had no change on him that day. Naturally this was all reported to the aunt and we were well scolded for asking for money. You must NEVER ask for money. And so we learned that lesson. But next day Toto came into the nursery with two bits of blue and white paper in her hand. "Mr. Fort has sent you a 1/- postal order each," she said and then she had to explain just what a postal order was to two excited tots who had never seen one before. So scolding had been worth while after all—until we found we had to put it all into our money boxes!

Toto had a mania for saving, inherited from her mother. Money would only be "frittered away" if it was left outside a moneybox—or the bank. It must always be kept for a rainy day. And she lived on this principle all her life and increasingly so as she grew old, so that when at the age of eighty six she had a fall and fractured her femur and when she was taken to hospital she was thought to be a pauper—until my brother flew over from Ireland to see to things. I was at sea at the time and could do nothing. But all the Dillons were the same; they lived in poverty and died worth capital in the twenty thousands.

Our next excursion into finance came after we had learned to write at least capital letters. We had often been to the bank with Toto and seen her give a bit of paper to the man behind the counter on which she had written how much money she wanted. If she could do it why couldn't we? In the nursery one morning when we knew she was going to the bank, we tore a sheet out of an exercise book and halving it we wrote I WANT SIX PENSE PLEES. With these hidden in our pockets and hugging our secret we followed Toto in through the door of the National Provincial Bank. She put her piece of paper down and was counting the result when, standing on tip toe so that we could see the man over the top of the counter, we pushed out bits of paper towards him as far as we could reach. The man smiled and picked them up. "What's this?" he asked and grinned as he read them.

"What is it?" asked Toto, putting her purse away. She took our cheques from him and looked at them. "You silly children. How can you be so silly?" she said, quite annoyed. "Come away at once." And taking one in each hand she dragged the silly children out of the bank while they were

tearfully saying: "Well, you give him a bit of a paper and get some money."
It seemed banking was not so simple as it appeared.

Scooters and hoops, large wooden ones which you bowled along, were
our main outdoor toys, but the chief delight of the summer evenings was
the gardens where we joined up with other children, except those who
didn't "speak nicely," that is, the children of housekeepers or cooks in the
various residences. (This was always the bugbear of the aunts, and accounts
for my present immediate adverse reaction to impure vowel sounds which
I have never been able to shake off.)

My chief friend was to be a boy of my own age called Tony Bentine,
who had a young brother still in the high chair stage who did not come
out to play but whom I saw when I went to tea in their nursery. Michael
Bentine at the age of one year had a mass of golden curls; now he is the
dark haired radio comedian of whom I have read but whom I have never
seen since those nursery days.

Round the garden path ran the bushes and here we had a house in the
trees and when half a dozen had collected we played either at homes or
schools, or climbed the lower branches and tried to swing like monkeys,
upside down. Tired of this, there was always hide and seek and, when old
enough, cricket, despite the notices that said prams, carpet-beating and
cricket on the grass were strictly prohibited. The gardeners had little
chance when we were out in full force and wisely kept to tending the plants
that were damaged by balls and feet.

On fine summer mornings too, there was the beach and the sea and the
rocks if the tide was out. This too was a never-ending source of pleasure.
I loved the sea. I still sometimes dream at night that I am going back to it,
despite my renunciation of the world. By the time I was five I had learned
to swim. This was due to the good offices of our cousin Auntie Daphne,
who was a keen swimmer herself and who then still lived in Folkestone. A
couple of years later she decided to break away from her family and live in
Italy where she first went to have her voice trained as she had aspirations
towards opera. But her voice, though good, was not strong enough and
finally she made a living by giving singing and English lessons. Then she
came home only for two months each summer, for her home life was not
congenial to her.

Aunt Daphne had the happy thought of buying me some water wings
to learn with. At first, however, I feared to trust myself to them and would
only walk up and down holding them round my waist. Then I fell over a
rock one day and found I was buoyed up, so took a few strokes and lo! the

first hurdle was surmounted. By the end of that summer I could manage without them.

The rocks were just as exciting as bathing, since they ran out for about two hundred yards, the ones nearer inshore being dry and having pools where there were shrimps and crabs to be fished for, and the further ones slippery with green or brown seaweed. On the dry ones you could leap from one to the other and perch aloft on a high one and pretend you were on a desert island for a few moments and king of the castle. Yes, Folkestone was a good town to grow up in!

At that period it was divided by an imaginary but no less real line into West end and East end. And on Sunday mornings after church there would be a regular parade on the Leas, that grass promenade on the cliffs above the sea, and the "gentry" would parade on the West end and the "town" on the East, and the limiting line would be second bandstand by unwritten law. Nowadays the line has gone: the Second War erased it, and West and East mingle freely at both ends.

With winter neither sea nor gardens had any appeal; but winter meant Christmas with all the excitement of that day of days, and also the pantomime and the Christmas parties.* These latter would be held by those fortunate mothers who had big houses and sufficient staff, for they were no mean affairs. The best and most popular of the year was that given by a Mrs. Dalison, whose only son was grown up but who was so fond of children she still gave this annual treat. And she was reputedly a wealthy woman. Her husband, Colonel Dalison, kept well out of the way that day.

The table would be covered with every kind of cake, jelly and sweet meat. At each place, which would be named, there would be a gas balloon rearing up to the ceiling, and after the tea there would be a treasure hunt, with three or four presents for each child. Indeed it was the party of parties.

At some stage about now I developed a strange and unfortunate allergy to sweet stuff, strawberries and chocolate. The allergy was physical, not psychological, for if I ate even one iced cake, the next day I would be out in spots, appallingly itchy, and which soon turned to massive blisters spread all over my body. I could no longer even have the evening sweet. So I would go to a party and gaze at those beautiful cakes and the hostess would

---

* In England, the "Christmas Pantomime" is a form of comedy play, traditionally performed around Christmas time, in which gender reversals and audience participation have historically played a prominent part.

have been warned of my idiosyncrasy and would have tactfully supplied a plate of sponge-cake in front of my place, and I would munch away, eyeing the pink and white and chocolate icings, but knowing that if I succumbed, next day I would regret it. Sometimes temptation was too strong and I would have a small slice and the inevitable followed. By this peculiar allergy, for the rash was not a typical allergic rash at all (and I have never seen the like since), I early learned the need of self restraint. When fifteen I went through a period of vomiting every week or two for three months till the doctor was called in and he took me off all sugar and put me on glucose for awhile. After that both rash and vomiting ceased and I could eat anything.

The week before Christmas seemed interminable. How could one ever get through it? Yet Christmas Eve would come at last and the letter to Father Christmas would be written and put in the fire to fly up the chimney to him. Once Granny, thinking I was throwing away a bit of paper crushed it down with the poker and reduced me to tears of despair, for now how would he know what I wanted? But Toto assured me that he would. It didn't really need to go up the chimney. And one year I left him a few sweets as he must be hungry after his long journey, and I was thrilled to find a note where they had been, saying "Thank you very much. Father Christmas."

The stockings were far and away the best part of the day. We never managed to stay awake, nor even tried to, so far as I remember, but hastened to sleep to make next morning come more quickly. Then in the dark we pushed our feet down to the bottom of the bed and heard the rustle of paper and squirmed in delight. When Nanny could be prevailed upon to put on the light (for it was gas in those days, no electric light switches), we would open those stockings and compare contents. For everything had to be the same for the first three or four years of our lives, so jealous were we of each other.

After breakfast we would undo presents, these would be piled on the cane sofa in the dining-room, Bobby's wrapped in blue paper and mine in pink, and it seemed as if there was a mountain of them. Unfortunately because of Toto's predilection for putting away all toys that were "too good to play with because they might get broken" the aftermath was greatly reduced. Forty years later, while clearing out the house after her death, I came across a curious kind of doll in a drawer and asked Daisy whose it was. She told me it was mine; it had been given to me one Christmas but Toto had thought it too good to play with so she had put it away—and I was a middle-aged man before I saw it!

But dolls held no interest for me and my fifth Christmas was unforgettable because it was such an unhappy one, the unhappiest ever until the War years when I had to pass two with no one and nothing with which to celebrate.

But this one was when I was five and the cause of it was Auntie Daphne who otherwise was such a kind "aunt." Her presents we always regarded as being the best of all and on this Christmas Eve she brought into the nursery two packages, one in blue and one in pink paper and at once they were whisked out of sight. In vain we begged to know what was in them but we were driven off to bed with no more satisfactory an answer than that one was for a boy and one for a girl. Next morning, after breakfast, we made a bee-line for these out of all the packages that were on the sofa. Bobby tore off the wrapping from his and revealed a pair of hair brushes, just like a man's. He looked a shade disappointed but said they were very nice. I opened my parcel and saw a small blue leather jewel case.

Bursting into tears of disappointment I threw it on the floor in utter disgust. That the best present of all should be such a stupid thing! Even Bobby's brushes were better than that. Toto picked it up and tried to comfort me by saying it was very nice and she would have liked it. "You can have it." I said ungraciously and turned to see if there was not some other treasure to compensate.

All might still have been well had not Auntie Daphne, at the family dinner to which all aunts and cousins except the Worthing one, came, asked us whether we had liked our presents. Bobby said, "Yes, thank you very much," although he did not sound over enthusiastic. She then asked me the same. Now it has always been a facet of my character to say just what I think or feel, a blunt honesty which has never been eradicated and which has often got me into trouble. "No," I now replied.

There was a sudden silence and everyone looked with horror at me and at once a dozen voices seemed to be telling me what a rude, ungrateful child I was and that I must apologize at once. But this I refused to do since, not only had I been grossly disappointed over the present, but I had been asked a straight question and I had given a straight answer. It being Christmas, I was allowed to finish the dinner and stay down but in direst disgrace for the rest of the day. Auntie Daphne seemed particularly hurt which she need hardly have been since I had only reached the tender age of five and had not yet learned polite dishonesty, and she said she would never give me another present until I did apologize. I stuck it out until a few days before my birthday some months later and when she was still holding to her promise, one evening I said I was sorry and as soon as she had kissed me and said it was all right I promptly climbed up on her knee and asked what she was going to give me for my birthday. By now I was learning diplomacy rather than honesty! But she, too, had learned her lesson for she never tried to give me a present "for a girl" again.

Boxing Day would be flat after all the excitement but the next thing to look forward to was the pantomime, brought each year for one week by Murray King, then getting on for eighty, so it was said although he still took the part of Widow Twanky himself. Never since have I seen a pantomime to equal those old-fashioned ones. Ice-ballets and flying troops [*sic*] and popular songs were small compensation for Widow Twanky's red flannel petticoats, the village school and the funny men who had much bigger parts than in these days. One feels that today pantomimes are actually intended more for the grown-ups. Sometimes we went with a party of other children and parents or grandparents, friends of our aunts. Once one bloodthirsty little girl of six at "Ali Baba and the Forty Thieves" kept crying out "Want to see Kassim cut up!" and would not be comforted because he had been cut up in the book and they would not do it to him on the stage!

We ourselves never had a party presumably because of the fiction that we were so poor. Indeed the only tea party in the nursery that I can remember proved a frustrating affair. We were told that our cousin Joan who had come from India was coming to tea with us and jam was put out and cakes bought. But when she came she refused to eat anything but lay in her nurse's arms and sucked from a bottle and she would not talk to us much less play. That was a silly sort of visitor to have, we thought. She had a white sun bonnet on and a long white dress, and I can still infuriate her by reminding her of the time she came to tea with us in a sun bonnet!

This was the sole occasion that we met our Uncle Joe, on his last leave before he died. I have only one recollection and that is of him standing in the dining room tossing Joan up and down in the air while she crowed with pleasure, and I wished he would do the same to me, but then I was too big being four.

Just when we first went to London to meet Daddy I do not know; Toto's aversion to travel limited my trips to one a year but soon Bobby was going quite often, perhaps with Maudie to escort. But I can only remember Daddy on three occasions.

To begin with he had bought a hotel, the Sorrento Hotel, at 6 & 7 Tavistock Square, now the site of the British Medical Association, oddly enough. He lived in the basement flat and had installed an Irish woman as manageress, an efficient business woman who looked after him well while having an eye to her own advancement. We were warned before we went that we might find Daddy ill and that he would not be likely to play with us or go out much. And sure enough, he never met us at the station but was always to be found in his dressing gown in an armchair in the basement flat. Later we learned that his "illness" consisted of hangovers.

The hotel was, like our Folkestone house, built round a public square but the central garden was much smaller than ours and no one played in it. Many years afterwards, when I once had occasion to go to the British Medical Association for a meeting connected with Ships' Surgeons, it was strange to walk again around that same square and look across at the same houses I must have seen as a child. Number six was bombed during the war and afterwards the whole was demolished and the modern imposing edifice put up, yet walking up the stairs and along corridors, the area being covered was the same as when my little feet had tramped up to the hotel dining room for lunch or gone to see one of the regular guests, a young house surgeon named Dr. Nicholl, now, I believe an eminent Harley Street radiologist. He it was who taught me to play chess when I could not have been more than seven. He taught Bobby too, but after a few weeks of my insisting on playing every day with him he went on strike and I do not think has ever played since, whereas I have always been most grateful for those early lessons. Better still, however, Dr. Nicholl let us fight with him and as we had never had any male grown-ups for a rough and tumble, this was a special delight. The only other regular guest I remember was a man named Arthur Chichester, whom I disliked because he wore bright colored hairy tweeds and insisted on kissing me with a rough bristly chin.

On two occasions we did go out with Daddy, maybe more, but only these do I remember. Once it was to Regent Park Zoo where a monkey made the day a memorable one by snatching off my straw hat because it was decorated with a band of artificial buttercups to which it took a fancy. I rode on the neck of a camel then, too, whether on the same or a later occasion, and never again did I mount a camel until it was on Karachi beach along with the stewardess off my ship, since a man was hiring camel rides for one rupee a time as a man might hire donkeys on Brighton beach.

The second occasion was another excursion into the realm of finance. Daddy wanted to buy Toto a new carpet for her bedroom and we went to a big furniture store where one was selected in emerald green. Then Daddy started haggling over the price and managed to get something knocked off, leaving a certain sum and sixpence. For a long time he jokingly argued with the salesman over that sixpence but could not move him. Bobby and I, in deep distress, since Daddy must be very poor, looked into our little purses and went into a huddle. We had enough! Then we approached the arguing pair holding out three pence each.

"We will pay the sixpence, Daddy," we said . . .

But Bobby seemed to go quite often without me and it was after one such visit, when he returned in time for Christmas that he broke the news to me that Father Christmas was Daddy all the time! I was shattered and tried not to believe it. This was my sixth Christmas. But the evidence was indisputable. On Christmas morning there had appeared a paper decoration over the fireplace, showing Father Christmas filling stockings. Bobby had seen it in London only a few days before and Daddy had bought it. So there it was. Toto, tearfully appealed to, confirmed the sad tidings. Nowadays it is the fashion to think that children should be told the truth early on and not "deceived" (despite the mass deception practiced in all other spheres by mankind) but I would not have given up those few Christmases in which I believed in him for anything. After all, you have had the enjoyment even if there is disappointment to come.

Between Christmases and birthdays, sometimes exciting events occurred such as the "burnt house." A house a few doors up the road caught fire one night and in the morning we were disgusted to find that we had slept all through the excitement whereas the entire street, apart from us, had been out watching the flames. We told our Nannie just what we thought of her for all we could see next day was smoking ruins.

Then sometimes there were visitors for whom we had to be carefully dressed and on our P's and Q's, which meant our best manners. These would not be the same as the tea party visitors, for they would come in the morning and stay to lunch at which, of course, we did not then appear. One of these we were told we must be most polite to because she was very strict and didn't like rude little boys and girls. She was to be called Aunt Daisy and her name was Daisy Diz. Actually it transpired her name was Daisy Disraeli, for she was a great niece of Benjamin and she had been a girlhood friend of Toto.

On another occasion came our Canadian cousins, Maude Brock, widow of the General, and her daughter, Mildred. Mildred brought me a lovely present of what seemed a huge clockwork liner, called the *Lusitania*, she said, though the name conveyed nothing to me then, yet it sounded very grand. But after several outings on a string in Radnor Park pond where all boats were sailed, one day it met the fate of its namesake and sank in mid-ocean, or rather mid-pond, since I had hoped it would go right across without the string and its engines faded out in the middle and it slowly capsized and sank amid a welter of tears. For all I know it may still be on the bottom with all the other wrecks.

Cousin Maude was Daisy's particular friend and, indeed, at some time she went to Canada to stay for the summer and great was the upheaval of her departure, but it was a well-earned holiday for her who had so few pleasures.

Toto, Daisy and Maudie, who lived with us and from whom we learned to talk, we called by their names without any polite prefix of "Aunt," simply due to the difficulties of early speech. Those who did not live in the same house or who were far away like Auntie Kate, a quarter of a mile down the road in Earls Avenue, and Auntie Grace in Worthing, had the honor of being Auntie. Personally, since having been grown-up, I do not like the modern tendency of children to call adults by their first names in casual fashion, often encouraged by their parents; it is carrying the demands for equality too far. But then I have always been conservative about customs.

Nursery days were shortly to draw to a close. One day Bobby returned from his holiday in London wearing his first suit, a dark grey tweed with proper shirt, soft white collar and a tie. I burst into tears. People thought it was because I wanted a suit too, and it was explained to me that I couldn't possibly have one, but that was not the real reason at all. It was because I perceived the end of an era—the end of nursery days when we were Bobby and Baby, for now Bobby was to go to school and I would be left behind and I hated the idea of any change in circumstances. This feeling remained with me until middle age, almost, again and again it recurred as will be seen, and finally it was only broken when I went to sea and found that after making friends in one voyage and loving a ship, one would be shifted next voyage and have to start all over again. After the first voyage the desire to cling to the past was firmly put away for ever. Now I do not mind launching out into new expediencies. The future holds more than the past.

CHAPTER 3

Schooldays

The school to which Bobby was to go was conveniently situated at the end of the road and it was known officially as St. George's, but unofficially as either Mr. Darby's, after the Headmaster, or The Pink-Cap School, because of the pink caps with blue roses embroidered on the front that the boys wore.

My envy of my brother going to school was deep and lasting. While I continued my lessons with the governess, in the afternoons I would see boys going in crocodile to the cricket or football ground or out on their Sunday afternoon walk. Sometimes Bobby would bring home a friend to tea on Saturdays but then sisters were *infra dig* and I was not encouraged to play with them. One afternoon when I was standing outside the house as the file of boys passed with cricket bats and pads, and with Mr. Darby with his own small son, not yet properly of school age, in the rear, I summoned up enough courage to tell him I wanted to go to his school too, but he only smiled and said he did not take little girls.

But there were some compensations in the stories Bobby used to bring home of school adventures and the tricks of his form-mates. One of those who seemed to be most often in mischief was named Gibson. Not till a long time after was it revealed that his first name was Guy, and he was to become the V.C. of the famous Möhne Dam exploit.*

Cigarette cards were also a novelty.† Wills' series of Wild Flowers, No 5 being the first I ever saw, dirty and crumpled from Bobby's pocket, but as Maudie smoked, although her elder sisters disapproved, we were soon collecting and swapping and sticking into albums.

One day Bobby came home and recited *Amo, amas, amat*, I love, thou lovest, he loves, etc.; he had begun to learn Latin, and at once I learned that much too, and *mensa*, and from this very early start I always liked Latin and looked forward to the time when I, too, should learn it, and was later to show my *penchant* for the classical side altogether.

Then just after my eighth birthday I set out for my own first day at school, in the summer term of 1923. There was only one possible choice for me, the Brown School, or Brampton Down, as it was called, with its n——r brown uniform. All the other schools admitted the daughters of business people and even tradesmen but this one catered exclusively for young *ladies*. The school stood at the top of Sandgate Hill, as it still does, I believe, in an area then countrified, since we had to cross a field and stile to reach it. Later we were to live in a house built in that very field, but that was not for another seven years.

Before any child was admitted she had to be able to read and write. Not yet were the days when with state education everything would be left to the teachers and parents would abjure responsibility for any education of their offspring. The Headmistress was a Swiss, widow of an Englishman, and called by all, Madame. The Vice-Principal was six foot tall and inspired us with awe both by her height and her deep contralto voice, but she taught only music and singing. While in the first form school was only in the mornings and there was no "prep," so I still had to find my own amusements in the afternoon when Bobby was not there to play with.

Red Indians were very much in vogue at this period, with the classic Western silent films, *The Covered Wagon* and such like a huge success, and

---

* Möhne Dam was a German dam that was bombed by the Lancaster Bombers of the Royal Air Force, commanded by Guy Gibson, on May 16–17, 1943. The incident became known for its dramatic, real-time disclosure to English Prime Minister Winston Churchill, U.S. President Franklin Roosevelt, and Air Chief Marshall Harris.

† Cigarette cards were rectangular cards decorated with printed images that were included in cigarette packages both as brand advertisements and to stiffen the packaging. Introduced in the late nineteenth century, they were discontinued during World War II.

those children's weeklies which would now be called "comics"—*Tiger Tim*, *Rainbow* and *Bubbles*—were wont to give away the feathered Redskin head-dress every now and then.* Eventually I managed to acquire a bow and arrow with blunt brass tips which was my main delight. Daisy had also taught me to sew a little and to do chain stitch embroidery and with some assistance I made myself a Red Indian outfit, tunic and trousers, with a broad seam on the outside cut to look like a fringe. This was my most beloved apparel and when I came in from school I would at once don it and crawl round the floor with my bow and arrow looking for Palefaces (all of whom would be having their afternoon siesta). A little later when we had moved house and I lived in the sitting room and no longer had a nursery, I would use the broad arm of the settee as a horse and take a running leap astride it as the cowboys and Indians did in *Bubbles* or birthday-present books.

I was in the second form, after one year at school, when began that series of events which was to alter our whole lives and for the worse. First of all Granny died one Sunday. This made little impact however, for she played hardly any part in childhood curriculum; there was merely the empty bath chair in which Daisy had always wheeled her out and the bare space in the corner of the top step. On the other hand the event saved me from being "kept in" one Saturday afternoon for persistently neglecting my geography homework, it being a subject I always hated. On the Monday I knew it no better than usual and the punishment was awarded. Not that it would have mattered in the least, but that Toto seemed to regard all punishment as dire disgrace and would go on harping on it until one felt embarrassedly ashamed, so that I was in an agony of fear for when she would have to know. But on the Tuesday the mistress called me and said she had heard what had happened over the weekend and there must have been too much disturbance in the house for me to work so she would not keep me in after all. I marveled at my undeserved luck and went on my way rejoicing.

On the Wednesday afternoon we had the treat of a ride in a horse and cab, Jordan's cab, as it was called after the owner, for the family was to follow the hearse to the church and Granny was to be buried and everybody else but ourselves was crying because she had gone to heaven. But Bobby and I, with black bands on our arms, were very excited at the ride which was so rare a treat and as I peered out of the windows covered with curtains, I was impressed to see passers by raising their hats as we rolled along, a courtesy not often extended to the dead these days.

* *The Covered Wagon* was an American silent Western that came out in 1923. *Tiger Tim*, *Rainbow*, and *Bubbles* were all British comic books.

Thereafter the house was to be sold and Bobby was to go as a weekly boarder to school while Toto, Daisy and myself were to move further up the road and have a set of rooms in a boarding house kept by a respectable widow. This should have been the moment for Daisy to break away but the misguided sense of duty which beset her impelled her to impose on herself the task of "looking after" Toto who was supposed to be so delicate, and as the result she came to lead a dog's life for the next thirty or more years.

For Toto was extraordinarily difficult to live with as I, myself, was to find increasingly, as soon as I began to break away from her apron strings. Domineering, utterly selfish, quite incapable of imagining anyone else's feelings, and expressing her own freely without regard to the effect, and becoming more and more miserly, no one of the family but Daisy would eventually live with her. But Daisy developed a kind of cortical deafness, that is, a complete unawareness of what was going on or being said around or to her, unless her attention was attracted, and she lived in a little world of her own, the only possible solution to the situation. But as yet this was still in the future. Maudie decided to go and live at the local bridge club where she had been wont to play nightly ever since the war had ended, and, because of the fiction that she was poor, she took on the job of hostess, which enabled her to live there free, and as she was a very good player she was able to make a small income out of it as well as to be a sought after partner.

As yet there was not very much change. The gardens were still there to play in of an evening and Bobby appeared at weekends. It was now that my friendship with Tony Bentine ripened as my bow and arrow was a source of attraction to him and he had a fairy cycle which I began to covet but which he hated and was afraid to ride. One evening we exchanged and went to our respective homes triumphant. Alas, unreasonable grownups no sooner found out than we were bundled out again and met half way down the road where we were made to re-exchange, which we did sulkily. It had seemed an ideal arrangement but there was no arguing with grownups sometimes, especially as Tony had a father who was very strict with him and beat him hard and long, so he said, whenever he was naughty.

There was another little boy whom I disliked intensely. He was said to be a Belgian refugee and he lived next door and had a tricycle. One evening I was trying to ride Tony's fairycycle down the road when he elected to thwart my progress with his tricycle, turning whichever way I went. Finally, just outside Bobby's school I got off, laid down the cycle and went for my tormentor with both fists and we had a good set to, which was watched with interest by the boys from the school. Next day Bobby told me my stock had gone up very much with them because of the fight, although I do not think there was any certain victory to either side.

Soon hand embroidery gave way to fretwork, and later, carpentry and I laid aside the needle and refused to take it up again until I had become a bachelor medical student who had to repair his own clothing.

We must have been in the new home for about eighteen months when one morning a telegram came for Toto who always hated and feared them. She stood fingering it uncertainly and the thought suddenly came into my mind: "I wonder if it is to say Daddy's died."

Then Toto opened it and gave a little cry. "Your father's died," she said, trying to stifle her tears, and she came across and kissed me. He, of all, was her favorite and there was only one year's difference between them.

In due course we learned that Daddy had gone for a weekend holiday to the Channel Islands and had contracted pneumonia and died rapidly. Mrs. Hearne, the hotel manageress, had been with him and had brought the body back to London. Bobby was summoned from school and was very upset, but then he had been going to spend all the holidays with Daddy since we had left the old house, and I still only saw him for one week in the year, since Toto would neither go herself nor let me go without her. "You wouldn't like to leave me, would you?" being her way of stifling any desire of mine expressed in that direction.

It was already beginning, this method of playing on my emotions to get me to do anything she wanted. "You can't really love me if you want to go away from me," or "you know I shall be worrying about you all the time and that always gives me one of my bad heads," or "after all I have done for you, surely you can do this for me?" and so on. And over the next five years it was to become increasingly prominent in our relations.

We all went to London for the funeral and Bobby and I saw the body of Daddy which had been embalmed and looked like a white waxen image. Bobby started to cry, being genuinely moved, and I cried too, but only because he did, for I could hardly feel the loss much, but ever since I have hated waxen images in churches and the like. He was buried at Kensall Green beside our mother. He was only sixty.

It seemed that Daddy had invested all his money in rubber shares which were at that time at their lowest ebb and he had left Bobby two-thirds and myself one third of the capital or income. The hotel was to be sold and the first £2,000 was to go to Mrs. Hearne and anything above that to be divided between us. But worst of all he had left Mrs. Hearne as one trustee and guardian and Toto as the other. No two worse choices could possibly have been made. Toto had no head for business and refused to take responsibility and she would sign a cheque book full of cheques at a time and send them to Mrs. Hearne who was an excellent business woman without many scruples, as will be seen later.

Three weeks or so later there died another member of the family we children had hardly heard of. This was Sir John Fox Dillon, seventh baronet and owner of the family estate in County Meath, Ireland. The ancient house, originally a fourteenth century nunnery, had been burnt down by the Sinn Feiners three or four years earlier. They had come at night and roused the old man in his eighties and his wife and their elderly spinster daughter and ordered them out, but had added with true Irishism: "We don't really want to do this, y'know, but it's orders. We'll give you half an hour to get out what you want and we'll halp you," and sure enough they did, and a few heirlooms were saved before the house went up in flames together with Sir John's unique collection of coins and many good paintings and other family treasures. He with his wife and daughter went to live on their English country estate in Herefordshire. His was the last house that the Sinn Feiners burnt before they gave up the practice. It was situated but a quarter of a mile from the famous Tara Hill which used to be the center of all Ireland and twenty six miles from Dublin.

This death completed the upheaval begun by the decease of Granny. Bobby, now aged ten, had suddenly become eighth baronet, the Baby Baronet as he was promptly nicknamed at school. It was fortunate, so the aunts never ceased to say, that Sir John had lived just those few weeks longer than Daddy, otherwise he would have had the title and estate which was entailed, and death duties would have reduced us to real poverty, but by such a chance was the Government deprived of its many pounds of flesh!

Life now changed completely. Daddy had been against public school education and had not intended sending Bobby to one but now with a title it was felt that he must have this background and his name was put down for one of the slightly cheaper ones, Lancing College, near Worthing, from which Auntie Grace could keep a distant eye on him and have him to stay on half-terms.

Meanwhile what was to be done about the Irish estate? Mrs. Hearne volunteered to go over and see how the land lay. Since she was Irish born and bred she would be quite at home there and be able to know best what should be done. So off she went and wrote later to say that the old servants' quarters, a long two storied building, still stood and was habitable, but that the old house was in ruins. The Government would give but a paltry sum if there was to be no rebuilding but more if a new house was desired and this she advocated, meanwhile offering to take up residence in the servants' quarters to supervise things, and to this the aunts thankfully agreed.

Sir John, annoyed that his daughter could not inherit either title or estate, had left a clause in his will, providing an annuity of two thousand pounds a year to be paid out of the estate to his widow during her lifetime, which was to prove a tremendous burden on the young heir, and quite unnecessary since the old lady was well enough off without it.

Shortly after this, we left the boarding house and went to live in a flat above a shop in the west end of the town, although how this agreed with all the aristocratic ideas we held is difficult to know. Nor do I know why this step was taken unless it was because it was now felt that we were really poor, what with Daddy's rubber shares and the burden of the Irish estate, although Bobby's and my money were quite separate. Bobby was to continue boarding at St. George's and to go to Ireland for the holidays so that he might get to know the neighbors, the nearest of whom was Lord Dunsany and he lived about six miles away. What he suffered as the result of this was never fully made known for it was not until he came of age that the unscrupulosity of Mrs. Hearne's character ever became revealed to the aunts, and when they then demanded to know why he had not told them anything before, he rightly said that no one would have believed him if he had.

On the other hand for the next four years we all went over there for a fortnight in the summer holidays and on the surface all seemed well. It was a wonderful place for children to play in. Some three hundred sixty acres of fields, with a lake and a pond, a cave wood, which reputedly had a tunnel linking it with Tara Hill, and barns and stables and a hayloft where you could jump from a great height and not hurt yourself.

Mrs. Hearne had a grown-up son, called Tom, who used also to stay sometimes. And he it was who first taught me to shoot rabbits with a double-barreled sports gun when only twelve years old. This was kept secret from Toto who would never have permitted anything so dangerous and who was also sentimental about animals, sentimental rather than humane, as a future story will show. He tried to teach me to fish, for the lake and pond were full of trout but this I did not like as the hanging of a worm on a hook seemed cruel, as also the removing of the fish from the hook. After one afternoon I refused to go again. But shooting was different, provided you killed the animal outright and I used to enjoy this although the sight of a wounded rabbit one day which Tom had to hit on the neck with the barrel of his gun to kill, upset me very much for a time.

There was no horse to ride unfortunately for it was magnificent riding ground. Not long before, a doctor had recommended that Bobby should learn to ride to strengthen his erstwhile broken leg. But he hated horses although he had to do it. On the other hand I would have given all I had to have been able to learn, but the fiction of poverty prevented it. Lessons were 5/- a time for an hour. Later when I received more money at Christmas or birthday I started spending it this way and so did do a little riding but never enough to become good at it and, after I left school, many years were to elapse before I sat a horse again and then I had lost all riding muscles and only managed to fall off at the slightest provocation.

It was on the occasion of my fourth and last visit to Ireland that a significant incident occurred. Mrs. Hearne had decided to take in paying guests after the new modern house was finished, to eke out the resources of the estate. On this occasion there were staying three friends, one of them an old lady named Fanny Moody, who had been a famous operatic singer in her day. One wet morning I was picking out tunes on the piano with one finger and trying to sing to them not very accurately, due to my lack of ear. At lunchtime Miss Moody inquired who was the man who had been singing that morning. Now no one else in the house had. Indeed, there was only Bobby (whose voice did not break until he was seventeen) and the old man in her party. I said it was I but she would not believe it, for she said it was a man's voice. But in fact I had recently been finding it more comfortable to sing the octave below middle C and on that I had been playing that morning. Next term, when I returned to school, the long suffering six-foot singing mistress who had borne with my unmusical effort for so long, could no longer stomach this new bass effort and suggested that I might be more profitably employed doing "prep" during singing lessons, to which I agreed. At present, however, the voice-breakage was slight and did not affect me when I talked, and no one seemed to notice anything.

I was now in the Senior School having put off promotion thither for a year when I was twelve, for just the same reason as I had burst into tears when I saw Bobby's first suit. It would mean the end of an era—the era of being a Junior. For another year I managed to stay down and so came into the form in which were three of my schoolfellows who were to become my special friends and whose acquaintance I renewed some years after I had secured the right to live as my real self and not as society had hitherto directed. For they could be entrusted with a secret.

The flat I loathed. The shop owners, a draper and his wife, objected to any noise above them, and there was no garden and no one to play with. I lived with Toto and Daisy and did a little carpentry during the holidays in shop hours only, because hammering and sawing was anathema to the landlord. My stock also went down at school and some girls did not like coming to tea above a shop—or their parents did not like them to come.

Then came the year when I passed my fifteenth birthday and with it came a change for the better in every way. I took the first steps in emancipation from the enthralldom of Toto's emotional states: I acquired a pretended "father," and we went to live in a house of our own, modern and self contained with a big garden back and front.

Annually the school went on an outing to Dymchurch, that smugglers' haunt ten miles away, to celebrate Madame's birthday. There we bathed, played cricket on the sands and had a magnificent tea ending up with strawberries and cream. On this occasion something went wrong with the bus which should have had us back by six o'clock and it would not start. I sat in it and began worrying because I knew Toto would be worrying if I did not come back on time. Then suddenly it occurred to me how futile it would be if I were to go on all my life worrying because she worried. How would I ever get along like that? No! If she wanted to worry, let her! I would never again worry just because I thought she was worrying. And with this resolve came a feeling of great relief. I had cut the Gordian knot!

When the Rev. W. H. Elliot was promoted to being canon of St. Paul's there came in his place a new vicar, the Rev. C. S. T. Watkins, with his wife and two daughters, the younger of whom was also sent to Brampton Down and entered my form. He was six foot, with fair hair parted down the middle and brushed back and he was kindly and understanding. It was lack of understanding that was making my life so unhappy just then. Sex had not entered into it at all as yet although my breasts were beginning to develop a little, much to my annoyance, and I secretly wore a belt round them until a schoolfellow found out and said I might get cancer and it was very dangerous, so I reluctantly stopped doing this. But apart from that I had neither knowledge of nor interest in the matter.

But it was quite impossible then or ever to talk to any of the aunts about anything and hope to be understood. If I made something nice with my carpentry and showed it to Toto, I would receive a "Yes, dear, very nice but don't bother me now." On Christmas and birthdays no longer were there surprise packages to open. Toto would ask me what I wanted and if I suggested anything she would say: "I'll give you the money and you can go and get it for yourself. I can't be bothered." And it was the same with the other aunts. Toto, too, was an impossible person to give any present to; she seemed to have the idea that it was beneath her to accept anything and many a person was told she did not like what she had been given or did not want it.

Once when I was fourteen and with little enough money I spent over a shilling on a special present. I thought this time she really could not say she did not want it. For she was always complaining that her spectacles were dirty and this was a little leather booklet with a piece of chamois leather for leaves and inscribed on it was, "You can't be optimistic with a misty optic." The shopkeeper at Cross' knocked off the penny three farthings, since they were more than I had, and I came home with it wrapped in tissue paper and longing for next day, to see her reactions. It was her birthday, September 9. She opened it and said: "Thank you very much, dear, but I wish you wouldn't go spending your money on me." A few months later I found it in her desk still wrapped up in its tissue paper.

Once, she had perforce allowed me to go stay with a school friend whose grandmother she had long known and whose father was a clergyman and keen Oxford Groupist. I was away three weeks, an unheard of thing, and when I returned full of excitement to tell her of all the wonderful things I had done, I burst into the sitting room with a loud "Hallo!" and was greeted by a "Don't make so much noise, I've got one of my headaches." My inside seemed to disappear, and I went out up to my bedroom as near to tears as might be. Never again did I try to tell her anything, although she often complained of this very thing. Just how unreasonable can adults become?

Small wonder it was, then, that I developed a violent hero-worship of the new Vicar and I began to pretend he was my father and he, kind as he was, did his best to fill the post without making either his own daughters or Toto jealous. Nor is this latter as fantastic as it sounds, for her affection was of the possessive type and she hated my making any close friends. Indeed, she eventually gave me an inferior social complex by her oft-repeated, "No, you mustn't go round there again—you are only making a nuisance of yourself and they don't really want you," if ever I asked to be allowed to go to tea with a school friend more than once. As a result I began cutting people to whom I had once been introduced under the sincere belief that either they would not recognize me again or would not want to continue the acquaintanceship. This led to my acquiring a reputation for excessive bad manners by the time I was seventeen.

Another result of this possessiveness had been a mollycoddling policy by which I was supposed to be delicate and was not even allowed to play the dangerous game of hockey until I was thirteen and then only because other girls' parents made representations on my behalf. When after three years my hockey stick broke, we were too poor, it was said, for me to have a new one. The Vicar bought me one out of his own pocket and passed it off as an old one of his own. Similarly, she would not let me go camping with the school Guide company although I was an ardent Guide. After one term when the school was closed half way through for scarlet fever and I and two friends went in to collect badges in a big way, I ended by having all of my Gold Cords work done except the week's camping. Still, nothing would move her to let me go and it was a long tirade of emotional abuse of the type already mentioned, so I was left with my All-Round Cords and twenty-two badges and the First Class. The Proficiency Badges included Boatswain's from which I was to derive much pleasure in later years!

But often I could get my own way by sheer repetition, and thus we came to live in that brand new house which had been built with three others on that very ground which had had the stile on the first day I went to school. It was a charmingly designed house with a wavy path up to a front door which had a rounded top like a church door. You went into a hall in which there was a brick fireplace and parquet floor, small though it was, and the end of the banister had a huge brown ball on it. The back garden was large enough for a tennis court although we did not have one there—it was divided into half garden and half vegetables, still leaving plenty of space to play. I also secured a tiny shed where I could carpenter without disturbing the two aunts during their after lunch nap, since the suggestion that I might like to sleep in the afternoon, too, met with but cold response.

But I still hated the holidays and liked school terms, since then there were others to play with and talk to. When not at school I had to go for walks alone since beyond shopping each morning the aunts hardly went out. I now began to long for some animal to take out and secretly bought two white mice. The Vicar allowed me to keep them in a cage in his garden and I would go down to feed them and take them out for walks on my arm. But after only a week Toto found me taking a little milk and a crust and at once wanted to know what for and then accused me of stealing and insisted on my taking them back to the shop. Then the Vicar allowed me to take his little rough-haired terrier out for walks. It was called Jinks but in time it died for even then it was quite old.

Toto herself adored cats and always managed to have one somehow. In this house she acquired a stray ginger, a doctored cat, which she said was therefore highly nervous and therefore must be petted and cosseted like an invalid. In fact she was shifting to the cat all the possessive affection from which I was trying to escape.

One day I saw a tortoise walking sedately along the very middle of the road and since it might be run over and did not seem to belong to anyone I picked it up and took it home, intrigued by the fact that it had a tail. The gardener, consulted, said it was a water tortoise because of its tail so a saucer of water was provided for it but no basin was allowed in case it drowned itself. It lived for the summer in the garden and when autumn came tried to hibernate in the flower bed. But Toto each time searched for it and dug it up again and put it out on the grass in the genuine belief that it would be smothered if it went underground. After two such attempts it died, whether of exposure or frustration was never ascertained.

Although Aunt Evie with Joan and Leslie had come to live in Folkestone a few years before, as yet the gulf in our ages was too great to make us children of much interest to each other. Leslie went to St. George's which Bobby had now left, and Joan to St. Margaret's, another girls' school nearly but not quite as exclusive as my own.

So as a result of life at the flat I had long since become an omnivorous reader. After my period with Tarzan of the Apes had exhausted itself from sheer rereading and had been manifested by a prolonged effort to develop my muscles by all kinds of exercises and extra time spent in the gymnasium, and Ballantyne was also receding with Henty,* I turned, under the influence of my hero-worship of the Vicar, to books on theology.

But this was not wholly due to the Vicar's presence. For a year past there had been stirrings in my mind of a curious nature which no one seemed able to understand if I tried to talk about them. The utter uselessness of the lives of the aunts and of their friends was puzzling me and causing me to ask the question: What is the purpose of life? What are we here for? Very soon it became specifically: What is the purpose of *my* life? Shortly afterwards I was contemplating the problem of how one could say what one had done to justify one's existence if one was on the point of death. This was to be the first sign of that driving desire to *know* which was going to pursue me for the rest of my life. In a few years I was calling it the Search for Truth and it went through many vicissitudes before I found myself anywhere near an answer.

When I was in my sixteenth year it was suddenly discovered that my knowledge of sex was woefully non-existent. It was the Vicar who made the discovery as the result of rashly asking his confirmation class of which I was a member, whether anyone had any questions to ask about anything in

---

* G. A. Henty (1832–1902) and R. M. Ballantyne (1825–1894) wrote historical fiction targeted mainly to adolescent boys.

the Bible that puzzled her. Now indeed I had! I had been carefully reading through the whole of it again and one verse had stuck in my mind as being excessively unjust and I could not understand why it should have been a law. It came in Exodus and ran thus: "He that lieth down with beasts shall be destroyed" (Exodus 22:19). Now I had lain down on the floor beside the cat. What harm was there? So up went my hand and I asked my question only to cover the Vicar with confusion. He told me he would answer that one later—which he never did. Instead he must have gone off to see the Vice-Principal, now the Head, since Madame had died, with the result that I was called to her study one day and told all about the bees and the flowers, the point of which, quite unrelated to lying down with beasts, eluded me. I never did like botany anyway! Then she gave me a book the Vicar had bought for me about more bees and more flowers, and I got tired of it before half way through and never finished it, preferring theology and Bull Dog Drummond, who was my current hero, while never having abjured the *Gem* and *Magnet*.*

The next year I began to teach myself Greek, partly because the Vicar knew it and partly because I had natural classical leanings. But there was to be no money for regular tuition, since although there was a mistress who could teach it, it was an extra. So I borrowed *First Steps*, [by] Ritchie, from her, an exact parallel of our Latin Grammar before we graduated to North and Hillard, and next Christmas the Vicar gave me Sonnenschein's *Greek Grammar* and helped me with exercises when he had time.

School Certificate year was now looming ahead. We were to take the Senior Cambridge in the summer of 1932 and needed five credits and two languages for "Matric." For that summer term I had to abandon the Greek therefore and concentrate on other subjects. History and Geography were my weakest, and the Georges were a dull period.† But we were allowed to do questions from any two periods and in my first years at school we had a succession of history mistresses who, therefore, all began again with William the Conqueror, who was much more interesting. So saying nothing to anyone I mugged up this period and sat the exam doing half the questions from each. When the results came out I had five credits and a Good,

* *Bull Dog Drummond* is a detective novel published in 1920 by "Sapper," a pen name of H. C. McNeile. *The Gem* and *The Magnet* were serialized stories, published from the early twentieth century until the beginning of World War II. They featured the adventures of schoolboys at fictional public schools.

† By "the Georges" Dillon/Jivaka references the so-called Georgian era of English history, marked by the reigns of the Hanoverian kings George I–IV, who ruled from 1714 to 1830.

the latter in Latin, but history and, *per impossible*, geography, had been conquered. But I had failed French, a language I hated since it seemed so cissy. Now I still needed another language. After much argument I was allowed to stay on and sit for Greek as a subsidiary at the end of the Christmas term. Better still, I was given tuition in it. Then the credit in Greek emerged and Matric was assured.

Now Toto wanted me to leave school. But when I asked what she expected me to do with my life it transpired her idea was that I should go shopping with her each morning to carry the basket and later find a nice husband of good family, of course, and enough money. Now I had developed an ambition of my own. Thwarted when I had suggested going to a girl's public school like a school friend who went to Wycombe Abbey, this time I had firmly made up my mind to get to Oxford by hook or by crook.

With no desire to leave school yet and so have no companionship, I tried to persuade Toto to let me stay on and do Higher Certificate. At first it was a case of not enough money, and so well did she manage to convince people of her struggling poverty that the Head suggested I stay on for one year free provided I help with the juniors. Having already suffered the indignity of make shift school uniforms throughout, this did not matter much and I readily agreed and so did she, for our aristocratic self-respect did not seem to matter when it was a question of money. This was in 1933. Years later when I was turning out the house after her death I came across her bank receipts for the year 1939. Her current account balance then stood at 1,900 odd pounds. So six years earlier she could hardly have been so poor she could not afford ten pounds a term school fees.*

Then occurred an event which I thought nothing of at the time although the first pangs were coming into prominence. There was a math mistress who was very attractive even in her college blazer and skirt which she wore daily for teaching. Her great friend was the history mistress who was a boyish, athletic type. At the end of that Christmas term the staff gave a play and these two were hero and heroine respectively. Next day the history mistress, Miss B., came up to where I was talking to some girl and said jokingly, "Well, did you fall in love with me yesterday?" She had been well attired in a blue suit for the stage. The girl I was with only giggled but I was frankly puzzled. "Not you," I said emphatically, "with Miss A.," and

* Hand-added comment by Dillon/Jivaka here: "And as a result of my methods with the Juniors a mistress told her one day I had been nicknamed Mr. Dillon by them—though I had not heard of this myself."

indeed, in a flowered frock and straw hat, on the stage she had moved me considerably. Quite unaware of the flutter that was to start in the Head's study when this speech was reported, I went on my way, still much enamored of Miss A. When her engagement was later announced I was highly indignant and became the butt of the fifth and sixth forms who ragged me for wanting to marry her myself. But still no one explained anything to me and I never realized there was anything unusual in it. To assuage my feelings I made her a book-trough for a wedding present.

There were some three or four girls going in for Higher Certificate and it happened that the Latin mistress fell ill so that the Head had only one recourse, to farm us out to a tutor who lived nearby, an old inhabitant of Folkestone who was well known as a University and Army crammer. His name was Mr. Whyte. While kind as he could be, underneath he had a tongue, doubtless developed for dealing with stupid and lazy youths, but scarcely suited for the ears of young ladies, since "bloody" was one of the chief words in his vocabulary, although he avoided the obscenities.

To him, therefore, we went, his wife warning him to be very careful. And from that beginning grew a friendship for which I can never be sufficiently grateful. But for him I doubt I should have ever passed into or through Oxford.

It was due to him and the Vicar with some help from the Headmistress who had long since decided that I had brains when I liked to use them, that the shift from the idea of taking Higher to that of taking Oxford entrance came. None of the three wished to see me touting the shopping basket instead of studying further. And both the Vicar and Mr. Whyte were old Oxford men. Could I get a scholarship? The women's colleges had but few to give and were restricted even in their places because of the demand. My Greek was insufficient for scholarship standard in classics. On the other hand my wide theological reading made that a sound possibility, since few offered theology anyway, although what exactly one would do with a theology degree was not decided. I had some idea about being a deaconess, although it seemed one could progress no higher than that in the church. My desire to be a missionary, which had been strong at the time of Tarzan's popularity, but only as a means of going to Africa, had no support from Toto, despite how much store she set by going to Church, reading the Bible and saying her prayers for a quarter of an hour morning and evening. Still, offering this subject would be the easiest means of securing a place. So I sat for a theology entrance, and became well versed in the problem of "Q" and the synoptic gospels, and the history of Christianity while continuing my Greek with the Greek New Testament.

But before I sat the examination I had a shattering experience which made me look at life quite differently from how I had been looking at it. Of course now that I was growing up I had begun to suffer from the naggings of all the aunts and grown up cousins, for not becoming womanly. When I was small, being a tomboy did not matter, I was told, but now I should try and be a young lady. It ran off my back like water off a duck's, for this criticism seemed quite unrelated to me anyway.

Then one afternoon I was out for a walk with the eighteen year old nephew of the Vicar who had gone up to Oxford the term before. We came up the cliff from the sea and somewhere there was a gate which he opened and stood aside to let me pass through first. Suddenly I was struck with an awful thought, for no one had done this for me before. "He thinks I'm a woman." It was a horrible moment and I felt stunned. I had never thought of myself as such despite being technically a girl. I finished the walk in silence, the silence of despair, and he never knew what he had done to upset me. But life could never be the same again. People thought I was a woman. But I wasn't. I was just me. How could one live like that? With no one to ask I brooded long on this at nights in bed, while still working hard all day—too hard as it turned out.

At length I went up to Oxford for the examination. An ex-mistress from Brampton Down who had first fostered my later keenness for writing, looked after me although I stayed in digs. And the day the examination was ended I fell ill, with a high fever. Unwilling to stay on with strangers, sick, I forced myself down to the station and on to the train sending a wire to Toto to meet me and arrived back in Folkestone with a temperature of 104°. I lay in bed for a week eating nothing and with strange mouth and face ulcers. There being no antibiotics in those days, only local remedies could be supplied and the doctor was quite at a loss for a diagnosis, but still he pulled me through. Some weeks later I heard I had been awarded entrances both at St. Hugh's and the Non-Collegiate Society, known then as Oxford Home Students (because one lived in digs) and now known as St. Anne's College.* But there was no scholarship. Pressure being brought to bear the aunts decided to pay the fees between them for the latter, which would be cheaper, so Toto, Daisy and Maudie added to my own small income inherited from Daddy of about £120 a year.

At last I was to be an Oxford undergraduate!

---

* The Society of Oxford Home-Students was founded in 1879 and became the St. Anne's Society in 1942. It was officially received as a full college of Oxford University in 1952, then as a women's college. It began admitting men in 1979.

CHAPTER 4

Oxford

Home turn the feet of men that seek,
And home the feet of children turn,
And none can teach the hour to speak
What every hour is free to learn.
And all discover, late or soon,
Their golden Oxford afternoon.

—GERALD GOULD

Someone has truly said that if you mention the word "Oxford" to an old Oxford man, wherever he may be in the world, at once a faraway look comes into his eyes and he becomes silent with a half smile playing on his lips. How true this is! Oxford exerts a hold on her sons forever afterwards and a bond is wrought between them all, which neither color, race nor creed can disturb. Once I met a Lincoln man on the island of Mahé in the Seychelles, and an L.M.H. woman in Hong Kong, an Oriel retired Hindu judge in Sarnath and a Hertford Sikh in Delhi—it was always the same, reminiscences of mutual acquaintances among lecturers and professors, anecdotes of sport and rags and the like. Oxford was ever the theme.

That summer, after I had recovered from the illness, Mr. Whyte set about coaching me for Pass Moderations which I would take in my second term before starting Theology, and this required Aristotle's *Poetics* in Greek amongst other things. Daily I went to him after lunch for an hour and learned much besides. And whenever I met an acquaintance it was with pride that I said as casually as possible that I was going up to Oxford in October.

And at last the day came. Toto saw me off at the station insisting that I sit in a lady's carriage, "for safety" and from which I extricated myself at the earliest moment. Then in a few hours those famous gasworks hove in sight after there had been but a passing flash of the towers and spires, and there we were drawn up in the station.

Oxford! Even now when I am supposed to have renounced the world and to have become detached from worldly pleasures, the thought of Oxford still has the power to move me. Not that my four years there were all a bed of roses, seeing that circumstances were what they were, but the charm of Oxford itself was lasting and the atmosphere of days gone by have lingered to attract the newcomer. I gleaned from her what she had to give despite all adversity and made a lifelong friend of a man who began as my tutor.

The Non-Collegiate Society which I had joined had a headquarters in Parks Road and its undergraduates lived in lodgings. By the way, never refer to Oxford men as "students." The only students at Oxford are the Students of Christchurch, that is the Fellows of that college, and the term "undergraduette" never found favor. We were, all of us, undergraduates. This Society had its own tutors but fortunately the classics don became ill and those requiring her services were "farmed out." This led ultimately to my being sent to that tutor who was to become a lifelong friend, but that is anticipating somewhat.

Something happened in my first term to produce a change in my ambitions. My private problems were becoming somewhat acute without advice or help, and I was introduced to Canon Tom Pym, chaplain of Balliol, not then quite disabled by the disseminated sclerosis of which he was to die within a few years. His name was well known in psychological circles and he devoted much of his time to the adolescent difficulties of undergraduates.

It was he who first advised me against trying to become a deaconess since, he thought, my motives might be suspect. What that meant I was not quite sure but a little later when I was discussing the project with "George" Cockin, the Vicar of St. Mary's, the University Church,* he came out with the same advice and added that I would be bashing my head against a brick wall.

---

* The text here has Cockin's name crossed out, but given how it appears a few sentences later without explanation or clear context, we are including it here. The same crossed-out section adds "now Bishop of Bristol, and who was never baptized 'George' but apparently was never called anything else, at least at Oxford."

Still only partially understanding, but since two people quite independently had said the same thing, I decided to take the advice and give up the idea. But then what about Theology? "George" Cockin suggested my reading Honor Moderations, first, instead of Pass, which would take five terms, and then see how I felt. So I went to the Principal of the college, the late Miss Grace Hadow, a woman of charm and kindness, and told her I wanted to change. She agreed in theory but was doubtful whether my classical background was sufficient. Indeed, it was not! The whole of the *Iliad*, the *Odyssey*, Virgil's *Aeneid*, *Georgics* and *Eclogues*, were expected as a mere foundation to the rest of the courses and one would have to be able to translate any passages set from these just as a start. Thereafter there were sets of Greek tragedy, Plato's philosophy and Aristophanes' comedies, together with equivalent Latin sets of books, then a selection of fifty books of Greek and Latin from which any twenty passages would be set and one would have to translate eight of them. Further there would be Latin prose and a special subject, and, since I would never be able to do Greek prose, a second special subject and an extra set of books, which was an alternative.

Today it would seem an impossible undertaking with my scanty knowledge of Greek. Euripides' *Alcestis* and Aristotle's *Poetics* were all that I had read and of Latin perhaps some five books. Somehow I managed to persuade everybody, including myself, that I could at least get a third class Honors, and so was given permission to try. When I returned for the vacation Mr. Whyte made a notable offer to my aunt that he would coach me free daily throughout my time at Oxford. To him I owe the fact of my M.A.

At Oxford there are three courses open to every undergraduate. To be social, athletic or studious. Of these he can do any two at once but no more if he is to be successful in one of them. On the other hand, Oxford's enervating climate demands that her sons take some form of exercise, and the all-studious ones are frowned upon even by their tutors.

For me naturally the social world was closed. I had long been finding it more and more difficult to dress in any sort of frock or go to a party where young men were politely condescending. But exercise I needed badly, and always have needed it to keep fit. In my first term I took up rowing and joined the Boat Club. In my second year I was stroking the crew, that position seeming to have been the one for which I was best fitted from character, weight and size. I was now 5 foot six inches and weighed nine stone four and still growing. On the occasions of our annual meetings, for we did not see each other more often now, Bob and I were in deadly rivalry over height, half inch by half inch one or other would have just become the taller. In the end I made it by half an inch but not until I had suddenly put on two inches between the ages of twenty five and twenty seven, and had reached 5'9", contrary to all expectations and textbook data.

Work and rowing: this was my life at Oxford. In that second year I became a Rowing Blue, yes, female students are awarded "blues" too, and was elected President of the Oxford University Women's Boat Club. Now up to then women's rowing had been something of a joke. There was an annual race against Cambridge and a race against London University, but the College authorities thought it was an unsafe sport for women who might have to bear children and they made it as gentle as possible. In my first year we were not allowed to row side by side, but each crew started off in succession and the race was timed. It was over only half a mile and had to be rowed downstream. Under such circumstances it could only be a farce in the eyes of true oarsmen. Further there was no proper uniform and feminine shorts of various patterns evinced themselves while the cox wore a skirt and no headgear.

As soon as I had been elected President I set about remedying all these things. The first important item was to secure a good coach and I obtained the services of an old Leander man called Danks who was a town crammer. By dogged perseverance and all my persuasive powers, for I had early learned the value of argument (indeed, my school reports had repeatedly said "Would learn more if did not argue so much" and the like), I slowly secured the changes necessary to make the annual race worth watching and to remove from the Boat Club its reputation of being a joke. That year we rowed side by side, the next we had the course extended to a mile and rowed upstream, on the Upper river, from the first bend to Godstowe we plied our oars while supporters ran or cycled along the bank shouting themselves hoarse, many of them from the men's boats clubs. Next day we had a magnificent write-up in the Sunday papers. At last Oxford women's rowing would be taken more seriously.

The psychology of dress being all important, as I discovered at the beginning of each year from the nervous reactions of would-be oarsmen improperly clad (since I was reelected President yearly, for the rest of my stay), Bukta Sportswear were approached and supplied cheap vests and shorts, white vests with blue at neck and blue tip to the short sleeve, and dark blue shorts and socks. And for coxes a proper cap, schoolboy in type with the crossed oars and O.U.W.B.C. on it. This could be worn by all who had won their "blues," the scarf for which was already in existence. Blazers and sweaters completed the picture, and the cox had white blanket trousers or grey flannels.

This, however, led to a regrettable incident and my first experience of the newspaper world which later was to become bitter indeed. We had bought a second hand boat, a racing eight, off Merton college and had to bring her up from the Lower River as she was housed in the O.U.B.C. boat house. Normally we did not row down there as the men insisted we keep to the Godstowe reach. On this occasion, as the cox was new and not very experienced, I decided to cox it up myself as the narrow passage by the gasworks might prove dangerous and I had often coxed for the purpose of coaching and was not too heavy as yet.

I went down with the others attired in flannel trousers, blazer and cap while they had their shorts on since we could not take much clothing with us in the boat. It so happened that the O.U.B.C. was having an outing prior to going to London to train for the Boat Race and a press photographer was down to take pictures of them. All unawares I stepped into the cox's seat and gave the signal to shove off our boat from the landing stage. It seems he snapped me just then. Next day in one of the papers, the *Daily Mirror*, I think it was, there was a photograph of myself in the cox's seat and it was captioned "Man or Woman?" and then followed a brief column on L. M. Dillon, President of the O.U.W.B.C. etc. Certainly with my cap, my hair being now more or less eton-cropped, anyone would have taken the photograph for that of a boy. And of course the aunts heard of it, although they favored the *Daily Express* themselves. Yet friends showed them the cutting and I received acid letters about making a freak of myself to which I replied equally acidly that I had known nothing about it and that I was in the ordinary wear of coxes. The fact that I looked more of a boy than most of them did was hardly my fault. They failed to agree!

In my fourth and last year, 1938 the O.U.W.B.C. reached its peak. We won every race of the year, against Cambridge, London, Kings, Bristol, Edinburgh, and then we went on the continent with a four to row at Amsterdam and Frankfurt regattas—not so successfully, for continental craft were different in structure. But at least no one laughed at the Boat Club anymore. After I left it fell once more upon evil days, unfortunately, and sent me an appeal for funds when I was a medical student which I could hardly then reply to. I do not know if it still survives. If it does may it remember that the coach is the all-important thing, the coach and the uniform together can make a crew out of eight individuals and a crew will win a race but eight individuals never will.

And in that last year, little did I know that just ten years from the time I stroked my last race for the Oxford University Women's Boat Club, I should be stroking the men's First Eight at Trinity College, Dublin while reading medicine there! In all the travail of my life this fact I have hugged most gleefully, that I was a women's "blue" at Oxford and then achieved my First Eight Colors at Trinity. Some compensations can always be found in life if one looks for them!

So much for the world of sport—what of work? I took Honor Moderations in my fifth term, struggling through the mound of texts, mostly with cribs and doing only the "spot" passages in Homer since there is a limit in this world of Time and Space as to how much one can cram into either. The Third Class Honors I had promised came up, were impossible, and with it such bad eye-strain from poring over Greek texts that for the next term I was unable to do any reading at all, by order for the ophthalmologist, and ever since I have been limited in how much I can do in any one day.

The two special subjects I had chosen were Greek Drama and Logic. And for the latter I was sent to the Philosophy tutor of Brasenose, the late J. I. McKie, or Jimmy McKie as he was always called. This was the lifelong friend I was to make. And it all began most embarrassingly!

I had been to tea with him and his wife at one of their Sunday afternoon teas for undergraduates and wished to return their hospitality. So, on the last day of term, after the Logic examination, I had arranged to meet them at Cadena café for lunch, in those days at 2/6 a head. What with the excitement of the exam or sheer absent mindedness, I discovered to my horror, when the bill came, that I had left all my money on the mantelpiece in my digs and I had to borrow from my tutor to pay for their lunch and my own. What embarrassment for an eighteen-years old! This was the beginning of a permanent friendship which proved to be of the greatest benefit to me when I needed friends most.

That examination passed, I no longer wanted to return to Theology but to go do "Greats," the natural second section of Honor Moderations in the faculty of *Literae Humaniores*. Logic had enthralled me who was always addicted to arguing, and to read philosophy seemed the obvious sequel. The college authorities were antagonistic since I had been given a place for a theology degree but once again by persistence and argument I won. Unfortunately for the next year Jimmy McKie had been elected Junior Proctor and would not be able to take outside pupils so I was farmed out to one person and another, of whom I remember only one, a French woman at L.M.H. who told the Principal that I was "brilliant in patches" and could get a 1st if I could read enough. Then at the end of his term of office once again I found myself back in the familiar rooms at Brasenose with the rudder on the wall which betokened that Mr. McKie had coxed the B.N.C. first eight in his own undergraduate days.

Philosophy was the next step in my Search for Truth and since the faculty demanded a course extending "from Thales to the present day" (which was 600 A.D. to 1938) one would imbibe the ideas of all the great minds down the ages. At least not quite all. In after years I was to ask my tutor how it was I had never heard of the philosophy of Buddhism during that course and he confessed he had never heard of it himself. Yet I was to find that the Mahayana metaphysics took the problems of Knowing and Being up where the Western philosophers left off, and went further than any others have ever done. But meanwhile there was much slow plodding to do before this vista opened up before me, a plodding which ever went in a forward direction seeking its Goal of Truth and often seemingly surrounded by darkness.

But for the moment I found the orthodox Western ideas satisfying while I studied the nature of Knowing and Being, theories of Truth and Knowledge, and the mystery of the unknowable thing-in-itself, while Ethics I made into my first subject, but not before I had returned to Mr. McKie, and that is anticipating.

For Greek History I went to Wade-Gery of Wadham, famous for his reconstruction of early Spartan history and much sought after both as a lecturer and tutor. Had I not gone to the Non-Collegiate Society I might have been confined to woman tutors all my days, but all we Greats people were "farmed out." By Wade-Gery I was accused of indulging in Socratic irony, since it was inconceivable to him that anyone *could* confuse the date of the battle of Marathon which I had recorded in an essay as being 480 B.C. instead of 490. Yet how could he know I had hardly heard of the battle of Marathon before that term and when I tried to tell him he would not believe it? Still, one essay on the Greek Tyrant Peisistratus was labeled "first class standard," but only one unfortunately. Certainly the French philosophy tutor's prediction that I would get a "First" if I could read enough might have been true but with the eye-strain which limited my reading, especially of Greek texts, it would be an impossibility. And there was still the whole of Herodotus and Thucydides' histories to cope with as well as Aristotle and Plato and Livy for Roman history.

Naturally, therefore, even if I had been socially inclined, there would have been little time for this. On Sunday afternoons in the summer we would punt or canoe up to Marston and beyond and take lunch or tea and of course, books, and in the winter it was a pleasure just to sit by the fire instead of going out on an icy river to ply an oar.

It was in my first term, however, before work loomed so large, that I felt the need to confide my troubles to someone in regard to dressing up for parties and not liking to be treated like a woman. At once she, a fellow and a graduate, wise in the wisdom of the world, said the explanation must be that I was homosexual. This was a new word to me and I investigated it and thought that she was probably right, but it did not occur to me that, even so, one did anything about it. This was left to that former schoolfriend who had gone to Wycombe Abbey, to tell me when I met her in her rooms at Somerville, for she, herself, it transpired was avowedly so. She advised me to take a woman and get over my repressions. This advice was to be given to me again and again, even by well known doctors, yet never did I take it. Somehow it seemed wrong.

This, however, did not prevent me from falling madly into calf-love, primarily with one of the coxes who closely resembled Shirley Temple of the films and was nick-named the Babe. Even so it went no further than my telling her so and she, kind and sympathetic, did her best to help within the limits of good conduct. Then she, herself, became engaged and my dream world crashed, although she admitted that had I been a proper man she would have been hard-put to choose between us, which was some consolation.

Nor was there any help during vacation. The moment I returned home I would be greeted with abuse for my short hair and coat-and-skirt attire, before even a question after my welfare. At last in desperation I thought to confide in Aunt Evie, who seemed a little more understanding than her elder sisters, at least in as far as she allowed Joan and Leslie more freedom than I had, despite they were younger.

I went over to tea with her one afternoon and began to tell her about my apparently being homosexual but before I had finished she had burst out into a contemptuous laugh and said I had been reading something and the sooner I got married the better. I cycled slowly away again in despondency. Was there no one who could understand?

Years later I was walking on the beach at Aden with my cousin Joan, when my ship had called there and I found her by chance off another ship on a round the world trip. For the first time we discussed our respective childhoods and I was surprised to learn that hers had been unhappy too, since it seemed that Aunt Evie was just as callous and unaware even of her own daughter's feelings as the rest of the aunts were of anyone's. And she told me that I could hardly have selected a worse person for such a confidence. Yet I had always thought that her twin, Maudie, was much harder in nature although not so bad as Toto. Daisy, on the other hand, at this time was wholly wrapped up in Bobby and had no time for me at all. Later, this was to change, but in the time of my greatest need not a single member of the family was of any avail.

But there was always the compensation of Mr. Whyte; how good a friend he was is hard to describe! Naturally I never discussed anything of this with him and what he thought I did not know but daily I went to him to cram up history and to debate philosophy. His wife had died suddenly in her sleep one night shortly after I had started with him and he led a very lonely life thereafter. When, therefore, I found out by chance that he was a keen chess player, I used to go round after supper once or twice a week to play with him in his flat and to be regaled with ginger wine and biscuits afterwards. That the aunts did not consider this improper might seem strange except that he was elderly and so well known in Folkestone and by now Toto had little control left over me.

At Oxford I came to make two friends of my own age. The first called Bill was a Teddy Hall Greats man on a scholarship from a Grammar School in the Midlands. I was still naïve about matters and one day when we had adjourned for coffee after lectures I suddenly burst out into full confidence of my troubles to him. He never batted an eyelid. What his internal reactions were I never learned, but he set about being a true friend and helping me in any way he could. With him I went to watch the Oxford University Boxing matches, to which women were not admitted, for which he went with me to buy a sports coat and flannels, and nobody ever looked at me twice.

Although not a skilled rowing man he turned out to be a good coach since he had the knack of teaching and I secured him for the Boat Club and he ended up by marrying No. 5 in the boat and having four children by her, thus upsetting the theories of the woman dons. In fact development of the abdominal helps rather than hinders parturition. It is the soft non-athletic women who have the hardest time.

To Bill I also told a secret I had kept for some time: that I had begun to smoke a pipe. This was due to my naïve and child-like reasoning that if any man should begin to take an interest in me, if he knew I smoked a pipe he would cease forthwith to be interested. So I forced myself through the early sickness stages until I came to enjoy it and never gave it up until the day I arrived in Kalimpong at the monastery gate. Then I threw it down the cliff, knowing I could smoke it no more.

The second friend, made a year later, was a girl who was in many respects similar to myself, and we developed a brother-relationship which did much to offset the need for companionship we both felt. It was with her at bow that summer vacation I rowed down to Putney from Oxford, putting up in hotels over night. The Club had a racing pair, that is, a coxless pair, made of 1/5 inch plywood and only sixteen inches wide. Control of these craft is of the highest standards of rowing and by the end of the trip we could do anything in the boat. There was the necessary affinity between us so that I could impart silently what I intended to do, put up the stroke, or paddle light or the like. When we reached Mortlake we then rowed over the boat-race course in reverse in one stretch, though I do not remember what our timing for it was.

With her, too, I took boxing lessons for one term from the University gymnasium instructor who was an ex-Army sergeant and intrigued by his unusual pupils. And once I went to the Judo Club for a bet, since no women were admitted, and luckily found only a single member there who showed me the first elements of that sport. Afterwards I told him who I was and his only comment was "Your voice doesn't give you away." In fact, when I had returned to Folkestone after my first term many people asked me if I had a cold since my voice seemed to have gone down another shade and roughened now for talking as well as for singing. But I had no cold and it stayed thus.

With all the clubs that the freshman is urged to join the moment he arrives up at Oxford, the only one apart from the Boat Club which I became a member of was one of the religious clubs, called O.I.C.C.U.* Having been bitten by an evangelist revival meeting at a susceptible age, a few months before I went up first, I resumed connections with evangelical groups, which were centered on the church of St. Aldate's, prominent in its attempt to interest undergraduates in religion. Opposed to this was the Oxford Group, then at its peak, but it failed to appeal to me and rued the day when it invited me to a meeting, since I insisted on speaking and then said that all through that afternoon I had heard a great deal about this and that person and his or her sins but the name of Jesus Christ had scarcely been mentioned. This was not at all well received, since it seemed the individual confessing all his misdeeds and thoughts was far more important!

With Jimmy McKie's term of proctorship finished I was allowed to go back to him. The tutors I had had before lacked his original approach with the result that my first essay failed to win any appreciation. He had asked me to write some 2,000 words on "Which is the Real Penny?" and I dutifully produced Locke, Descartes' and others' theories on the nature of the thing-in-itself and only met with a "I know what they said, what I want to

---

* OICCU stands for Oxford Inter Collegiate Christian Union.

know is what do *you* think?" So for the next week I had to write an essay of the same length on "Is Queen Anne Really Dead?" and now being free to speculate on my own on the soundness of knowledge that is not from direct perception, I did rather better. This was his line and nothing else could have stimulated my own ideas so much, while my reading was also being directed into suitable channels.

At some time, from whom I do not know, I heard the dictum of some unknown mediaeval logician quoted: *Causa rei est res ipsa.* The cause of the thing is the thing itself. Perhaps it came from Mr. Whyte, but it was thrown out without explanation. Yet it struck me forcibly as being a profound truth and many years later I was to find it as the embodiment of Mahayana metaphysics, and I felt quite at home with the Buddhist teaching.

When I came of age and ceased to have a guardian or trustee I found I still had about £120 pounds a year of my own, not enough to live on even in those days, but the arrangement with the aunts about my college fees remained and for the rest I looked after myself. That same Auntie Daphne who had caused so much havoc over my fifth Christmas now presented me with a heavy gold signet ring with the family crest on it and the day of my birthday inside. I treasured that ring and only forced myself to part with it when I had decided to take up a monastic career, and then simply because I was reluctant to. Through the war years when my social position degenerated so far, that ring remained with me as a symbol of what I really was despite the outward appearance of being a grease-monkey in a garage!

At the beginning of my last term I bought a motorcycle. It was a light 2-stroke, Coventry-Eagle and cost £17 and was the best bike I ever had. Knowing that it would be considered most dangerous if the aunts found out about it and that I would be badgered into selling it again, I said nothing in my letters home but decided to ride down from Oxford to Folkestone on it and that would prove conclusively that it was quite safe.

On the day I bought it the manager of the shop said he would send a man with me that afternoon to learn to ride it as I had never been on one before. By after lunch when it was time to go, the rain was pouring down. Nevertheless I arrived at the shop and a very reluctant salesman mounted the bike while I perched on the pillion and off we went on to the Oxford bypass out of the town's traffic. Then we changed places, or rather, at first he ran beside splashing in the puddles. After I had learned to change gear, to start and stop and accelerate, he decided he had had enough and took a bus back, leaving me to practice alone. And still the rain poured down and I had no proper cycling clothes.

Fed up with the weather, I decided I should have to ride it back some time so might as well start straightaway and so, without an L in those days,* I cruised towards Oxford and crawled carefully in second gear up St. Aldate's and dropped to first at Carfax, the center of the city and crux of its traffic and then turned down towards the station where the shop was situated, arriving soaking wet but intact.

The salesman, who seemed to have had something of a conscience about having left me, looked in undisguised admiration: "I thought you said you had never ridden one before," he said. "I haven't," I replied. But he did not seem to believe me. Actually it was similar to the sink or swim business when you are thrown into water out of your depth. I had to get back several miles and so had to ride the thing.

It was while I was at Oxford still, that Bobby's troubles began to be revealed. His relations with Mrs. Hearne had been becoming more and more strained, it seemed. And at last while he was over in England on his annual short visit to Folkestone, she sold a cow of his in open market that had been condemned as tubercular, writing to congratulate him on the price she had obtained. His letter back was stiff and to the point and the rift occurred. He next heard she intended selling him up completely and leaving Ireland for good.

When they had first gone over when he was still a child, it seemed she had bought out of her own money, so she said, a great deal of the furniture and fittings for the new house. At all events she had said nothing about this before. At that time she had social ambitions as guardian of a baronet, and while he was still young she was naturally invited by the neighbors to accompany him to parties at the other country houses round about. When he finished school he went to Trinity College, Dublin to read Law, and began to make friends of his own. Further she herself was of peasant stock and her conversation and actions were not always suited to her company, with the result that he began to receive invitations which omitted her. This was an end to her hopes. Hitherto she had him completely under her thumb and had tried to keep him a child for as long as possible. Whether her ill treatment was solely mental or physical as well, we never learned, for this was the first news we had of any rift between them, but he had been a nervous child and could easily have been tormented mentally; in fact I

* "... without an L" refers to a plate or sign with the letter L, for "learner," that is meant to be affixed to the front and back license plates of a vehicle or motorcycle driven by someone who has only provisional approval to drive. Speed limits usually accompany a driver under this restriction.

had suspected something like that on my last visit to Ireland when I was fourteen.

Be that as it may she was not bluffing and made arrangements to auction the contents of the house, omitting only a few articles which Daddy had bequeathed to Bobby and which she could not touch. Characteristically none of the aunts went over to try to interfere. They were utterly bewildered by this apparent *volte face*. But Bobby's neighbors all boycotted the sale, which was attended only by professional brokers from other parts of the country and she departed with the proceeds leaving him with one room partly furnished. And still the two thousand per annum had to be paid out of the estate as a result of the bequest of old Sir John to his widow.

But the neighbors were not so ignorant of what had been going on as were the aunts so far away. When I was myself a medical student in Dublin and on a visit to a friend in Belfast, his mother's father, I quickly learned, had been the trustee of the estate until Bobby came of age and they were relatively near neighbors and had known Bobby from the first, naturally. She told me that her mother had often said, "That boy ought to be taken away from that woman." But there was no one to hear her. Also he told us himself now that the denouement had occurred that an elderly man who had been a friend of Daddy and who lived with his two sisters in Ireland, sent for him when he was dying and refusing to have Mrs. Hearne in the room told the child to "beware of that woman, she is utterly unscrupulous." The effect of that declaration from a dying man on a nervous child can well be imagined, but still he had said nothing to any of his relations.

When Mrs. Hearne packed up and transported herself to England to open a hotel in Hertfordshire on the proceeds, Daisy went over to Ireland to help Bobby and gave him £100 towards refurnishing and sewed curtains for the rooms. She stayed a month and the bond between them was a close one, since Bobby had always preferred her to Toto since babyhood.

Poor Bobby! He needed a feminine frippery type of sister to offset his own lack of masculinity; for it had been said even in our nursery days that he should have been the girl and I the boy. He hated sports and although by no means could he be called effeminate, he enjoyed gardening, bridge parties, played the piano very well and could draw and paint, even as Daddy had been able to. His accomplishments would have been better suited to me as mine to him.

He did not approve of my Oxford career or of my rowing or of my short hair or mode of dress, and who can blame him? But I could not be other than I was.

The final examinations were over, the last paper written and only the *viva voce* to come sometime during the Long Vacation. This, if one's place was already assured, would be a mere formality; if one was on the border line between two classes, it might be long and searching.

On my last afternoon at Oxford I cycled slowly all round the familiar streets, down the High to Magdalen Tower, where, on the first of May each year, my birthday, my friends and I together with Mrs. McKie would go down to hear the Magdalen choir sing a Latin hymn to welcome in the spring at six o'clock in the morning. Up the Turl and round the Radcliffe and Old Divinity Schools out into the Broad, down the Corn and back again up the Giler—those odd perversions of their names that generations of undergraduates have given to the streets and roads of Oxford. Then off down the Upper River where I had been so happy rowing and along the towpath to Godstowe. Then I crossed Port Meadow for the last time as an undergraduate and sought Bradmore Road where Mr. and Mrs. McKie were awaiting me for tea. Next morning I left early on my motorcycle, my luggage sent safely and swiftly by railway in those pre-nationalization days.

Later I heard I had achieved a Third Class Honors, the best I could hope for under the circumstances. And I had found my golden Oxford afternoon!

CHAPTER 5

War—The Darkest of Days

In this next chapter of my life I was to reach the nadir of mental suffering, before the dawn broke and all my troubles resolved and I could live a normal life like everyone else. But for the moment I was a museum piece. If I went into a café and sat down for a meal when I rose to leave, persons who had come in after me would audibly voice a wondering: "Oh, I thought that was a man." I have sat on a seat in a bus and listened to husband and wife discuss openly to which sex I might belong. To pass children playing in the street became especially difficult. I would be certain to have ribald comments hurled after me. I developed a "poker-face" to it all, but underneath was sheer agony of spirit. A museum piece I was and it seemed I would always be so.

It may be asked why I needed to dress in a "mannish" way or have an eton-crop, thus calling attention to myself. It is impossible to explain to anyone who has not had the same experience, any more than he who has just emerged from the dentist's chair can convey to his friend what he has endured from the drill, when his friend has never been further than the dentist's waiting room. I could not do other than I did, while still abjuring any advice to "take a woman" and relieve myself of some of my repressions.

I left Oxford in 1938. There people who looked like me were not quite so rare. Then I went to work in a laboratory in Gloucestershire, where brains were being researched on, both pre-mortem and post-mortem, since the philosophical problem of mind and matter had fascinated me and it seemed logical that one should learn something about the physical basis of the mind, which philosophers so persistently ignored. Indeed, I was already becoming irritated by the superior attitude of the philosophic world to the scientific, as later I was to be equally irritated by the scientific world's contemptuous attitude to the philosophic. There should be a bridge between the two, I argued, unaware that two famous men, Jeans and Whitehead* were also thinking along the same lines and beginning to publish books to that effect.

I went to live in cheap working-class "digs," having my experience of such life for the first time, and there learned that the accepted code of manners of that said sphere differed much from what I had been taught. For instance, if you asked for something to be passed at table which you could reach by stretching your arm, you were just making a nuisance of yourself. And if you offered someone else something before helping yourself you were putting on airs. After Oxford "rooms" it was all very strange. My motorbike, extremely useful for going to work, was also a measure of relief since I could tear around the country lanes trying to get away from myself as I felt at the time, unaware then that one could never do so. But now that rowing was finished lack of exercise added to the toll. True, I got in touch with Bristol University's Women's Boat Club whom we had beaten the year before, and coached them, with the result that at their next summer's regatta, for the first time in their history the Bath Ladies had the surprise of following their adversaries instead of leading them over the course, since the Bristol women had had no coach before.

Happy in what I was learning, but utterly miserable otherwise, my thoughts began to turn toward effecting a change, but without much hope since medical science had not progressed far at that time in such matters. Once when I had been seven or eight in London, Mrs. Hearne had said jokingly, "We'll take you to the blacksmith this afternoon and have you

---

* This reference is to two British scholars: the physicist and mathematician James Jeans (1877–1946) and the mathematician and philosopher Alfred North Whitehead (1861–1947).

changed into a boy." And I had taken her seriously in my delight and excitement, only to be reduced to tears when I found that such a thing could not be after all.

The doctors at my place of work regarded me as a curiosity and the girl secretaries were friendly and kind but without understanding of the situation. Shortly before war broke out I joined the W.A.A.F.* territorials who met once a week to learn to drill and deport themselves like soldiers. Then from the day war was declared we were called up for full time service, although still living wherever we were until accommodation should be provided. As a motorcyclist I was detailed to be a dispatch rider, but ere a week was out the Commandant told me she did not think I was suited to a woman's corps, and when I learned I should have to sleep in a dormitory of women, an idea that had not struck me in my first burst of patriotism, I agreed. As it was in my overalls on the motorbike I was always taken for a boy.

So back I went to the laboratory to find the lab-man had been called up so [I] was able to step into his job and extended the scope of my work to that of postmortem assistant and radiographer as well as microscopic work in the lab itself.

Somehow I heard of a doctor in the town who was said to be an expert on sex problems and to him I went to seek advice. He was interested and wished to help, at first postulating that a psychiatrist friend of his be brought in to make it an official experiment. So to the psychiatrist I went in all good faith and answered all his questions but the next time I visited the doctor full of hope he had suddenly become afraid and, expecting his own call-up shortly, which might mean leaving me in a half-finished and worse state than before, he backed out and I rode back to my digs once more in gloom, but in my pocket were some male hormone tablets he had thrown across the table to me. "See what they can do," he had said.

Shortly afterwards the psychiatrist was spending an evening with a friend of his who was one of the doctors where I worked. Without regard to medical ethics he recounted to this doctor all that I had told him and in turn, the doctor repeated it all to his colleagues, and I learned of it from one of the secretaries. Instead of being merely a curiosity I became a joke amongst them. "Miss Dillon wants to become a man!" was considered extremely funny.

* WAAF stands for Women's Auxiliary Air Force. Started in 1939, it was the women's counterpart to the Royal Air Force in England.

Unable to stand it any longer I gave in my notice and then joined the F.A.N.Y.'s,* moving into digs in Bristol proper. The F.A.N.Y.'s had been deputed to drive the American Ambulances which had been sent over and which were stationed in a suburb of Bristol on the Downs while the drivers accommodated themselves in a luxury hotel a couple of miles away down by the river. On suggesting it would be more to the point to camp at the garage, at any rate for those on night duty, or to take over a nearby empty house, I was told that you could not expect *ladies* to do that, although as the war progressed they were to do much harder things and to make a good job of them. But as yet the war was hardly being taken seriously.

After a few weeks, while riding to the garage for my morning duty, I went into a front wheel skid on loose gravel which the Corporation had elected to put down on a bend in the road. The cycle veered across the road, up the pavement, hit a garden wall and rebounded into the gutter where I lay face down with the motor bike across one leg, pinned till rescued by a passerby. For some strange reason people who rush to accidents seem to think the first essential is to stand the victim on his feet. Once he is right way up he looks more natural, and I had to fend off those who were trying to do this until I was sure no bone in my leg was broken. As it happened there was nothing worse than a giant hematoma, that is a bleeding of the muscle tissues internally producing a great distension, pain and discoloration. It was a month before I could walk again properly and even then I was weak and shaky. But this gave me the opportunity of resigning from the F.A.N.Y.'s whom I regarded at that time as dilettanting with the war.

Money was running short since I was not earning and one day when on a bus in the town I saw an advertisement for a petrol pumps attendant, male or female, pasted large in a garage window. I left the bus and applied for the job, showing my driving license, for I had passed the driving test in my first year at Oxford. Not quite sure what to make of someone whose skirt belied the upper half, the boss nevertheless accepted me since the shortage of labor was acute. And so began my career in the garage which was to last for four miserable years.†

---

* FANY stands for First Aid Nursing Yeomanry. Having been founded in the early twentieth century, during World War II its work was mainly in transportation for medical and other military purposes.

† Added here by hand and then crossed out: "It was the worst period of my life."

On duty at 6:30 a.m. to admit the workers at the Aeroplane shadow factory, who wanted to park their cars with us, I had two hours off in the afternoon and then worked till 6:30 in the evening. That spell in the afternoons was devoted to a visit to the public baths where one could get a hot bath for 9d.—or was it 6d. I forget.

But the very day before I started work came the first blitz on Bristol.* Unheedful of the warning from Cardiff's Swansea's sufferings, the Bristol authorities had not made firewatching compulsory and a stick of incendiaries fell in Regent Street, the heart of the shopping center.

One shop without a guard had a Christmas card depot upstairs, with its Christmas stock just in, and the flames licked greedily at it, devoured it and then spread rapidly until the whole street was destroyed and neighboring ones attacked. The garage also suffered but there was a night watchman, an ex-Public schoolboy, Swiss by nationality, who had been ousted from the R.A.F. after the Dunkirk scare,† and he tackled an incendiary single handed and put the fire out but he suffered from the smoke and informed the boss [the] next day that one man alone could not handle a garage large enough to park one hundred cars. But no one was keen on firewatching and as yet it was not compulsory. Being in dirty lodgings, I thought I could be no worse off sleeping at the garage and being woken just for air-raids, and so I entered into an arrangement to do just that at an extra 10/- a week—but then no one knew just how intensive the raids were to become.

Christmas I spent alone, on duty all day, being the only one without a home to celebrate it in, and the firewatcher had given in his notice as he wanted a better paying job in a factory in the Midlands. Advertisements brought us no reply. Then the day before he was due to leave I was going to lunch when I saw across the road a fair, curly-haired boy of about sixteen or seventeen with rosy cheeks. On my return from lunch he was wandering round the garage waiting for the boss to come back. I began talking to him and he told me he had come up from Swansea where his entire ARP‡ post had been wiped out by a bomb while he was out on a message. Unwilling to remain he had come to Bristol looking for a job.

---

* Bristol, which was subject to particularly heavy bombing raids during World War II, was first bombed on November 24, 1940.

† The Dunkirk scare refers to the evacuation of allied troops from the French seaport of that name as the German army advanced toward it from lands it had captured in the south. The evacuation lasted from May 26 to June 4, 1940.

‡ ARP stands for Air Raid Precautions, a group whose purpose was to help protect civilians from air raids.

I suggested firewatching would pay better than day work—as a full-timer he would get 3–5 pounds a week. When the boss came back I took the boy to the boss's office and at once the job was clinched. That was the start of a strange friendship of two persons utterly different in every way yet oddly complementary. He had been brought up in Muller's orphanage in Bristol, it transpired, not knowing who his father was, and Muller's orphanage was a place of Dickensian horror until the corporation demanded changes after the war. His life might have been that of Oliver Twist although he had never read that book for his education had been scanty, and as soon as he was free of the institution where he had been underfed and overbeaten, he went down to Wales where the woman he called his mother lived with a selection of offspring who bore no resemblance to one another.

Now from the very first days at the garage my workmates had never lost a moment in telling every newcomer: "You see that fellow over there? Well, he's not a man he's a girl." And even the foreman of the workshop whose ear drums had been burst in the Great War and who had to have everything written down for him, had had this written too. I made no mention of anything to G.* until the day before he was due to leave after being called up for the Navy some months later. Then I asked him if he knew since he had never given any sign but always treated me as if I were another fellow.

"Oh yes," he said, "They told me the first day, but I told them I would knock the block off anyone who tried to be funny about you. I also said you really were a man and that had them puzzled. They didn't know what to believe then."

"A faithful friend is a strong defense and he that hath found one hath found a treasure." So said Solomon in his wisdom. My debt to G. for this loyalty in my darkest hour could never be repaid although I did my best in later years.

In the evenings in the garage office where we slept on the floor, I used to talk to him, or rather at him, in Oxfordian style, and he listened only half comprehending at what he was pleased to term a lot of "stiff-shirt nonsense," a phrase I had never heard before! But it made him think for the first time in his life, so he said many years later. And when anything had upset me during the day—and there was plenty to do so—I would let off steam at him at night and he took no offense or even any notice, knowing well what I was contending with.

---

* In *Michael née Laura*, Liz Hodgkinson identifies "G." as Gilbert Barrow.

With the rest of my colleagues I had nothing in common. Their code of morality was utterly different from mine, I found, and instead of understanding we mutually looked down on each other. After I had been serving petrol about a fortnight, one of the workshop boys came to me and said with a friendly grin: "I suppose you're making a good thing on the pumps." I stiffened at the innuendo and asked him what he meant.

"Don't you know?" he asked, "I'll tell you." And he meant it in a kindly fashion. "When the meat lorries come in you pay the driver a bob to sign for thirteen gallons when he has only had twelve and then you have one in hand to sell for double that." He was unprepared for the blast that followed. The whole of the sense of honor that was incorporated in my background rose and I fairly withered him with words. He backed away eyeing me suspiciously, and the thought was in his mind, "Perhaps this is one of the boss' stooges." We were mutually shocked, I by such a suggestion and he by such a reception of it! The point was that the Meat Wagons, under the Ministry of Food filled up in our place and the drivers were not trusted with the petrol coupons which were filed in the office, and then they would sign for as many gallons as they needed and the bill would be paid and the coupons sent in monthly.

I also discovered that if anyone "won" something belonging to a mate a terrible fuss was kicked up and the victim went whining to the boss. But if anyone stole anything from the boss or a customer it was nobody's business and no one knew anything about it. Customers were also fair game, no matter that they had to pay for the mechanic's time on a job; and the mechanic would think nothing of going off for a snack or driving a car he was delivering a roundabout way to visit someone en route.

During the next three years I was at constant loggerheads simply by trying to keep to my own moral ideas. And the boss reproached me for quarrelling with my mates. Once after he had blamed me for a row, I was sent out on a breakdown wagon with a lad who wanted to go and see his girlfriend, which meant a detour. I agreed, for the first time, and a tidy sum was added to the customer's bill in breakdown petrol and our time. Some weeks went by and the boss was once more on about my not getting on with the others, so I told him of the incident without saying when or with whom it had occurred but pointing out that had I refused as usual, there would have been another row. Then he did not know what to say. But this was much later, when, after the blitzes had stopped, I was promoted from the pumps to tire chief and breakdown driver and the boss had also begun to use me to deliver and fetch customers' cars because I "spoke nicely"! At first he insisted on putting a "Miss" before my name but customers thought they were having a rise taken out of them and became annoyed so he gave it up after a while and instructed the staff to refer to me as "he" to customers. I still remember the car numbers of some of my favorite customers. There was EHY 221 who was editor of the *Bristol Evening Post*, and GHW 8 whom I liked best of all and EHW 200 who was a fearsome drinker—but there—the cars must be on the scrap heap by now and where are their owners? It was all of twenty years ago.

In the cold and dark mornings of the winter I regularly opened up the great running doors to admit the Aero workers at the first knock. In haste they would drive in and leave their cars anywhere and take away the keys that they might not be driven and so waste precious petrol. The floor that had been burnt and was now covered with sand was their specific parking place and the cars had to be pushed, one arm through the window to steer, the other hand on the mudguard, unless the car and sand together resisted too much, and then they had to be heaved from the rear by dint of walking backwards glued to the back wheel. It was hard work but hard work suited me and my muscles, firm from rowing, became fuller and tougher, aided also by the hormone tablets which I continued to take and which began to make my beard grow.

Breakfast was to be had at the tea stall on the corner, tea and jam buns, and then all the morning there was car pushing, driving or sometimes minor repairs, but it was quickly discovered that I was not mechanically minded. Once, however, when labor was very short I de-coked a Morris Eight in nine hours and it went again, to my surprise as well as everyone else's, and I was taken to task by my mates for not having taken ten hours, the statutory time.

All this and I was awake many nights as well since the sirens began going regularly with the nine o'clock news. Within a week of G.'s arrival they became almost a nightly affair. Bristol was badly battered during that winter of 1940–1 which was bitterly cold and one newspaper bore a picture of an arc of ice extending from the nozzle of the hose pipes playing on the quay during a blitz.

Then with spring came that biggest blitz of all, on Good Friday, when Churchill was due to come to Bristol next day for a degree at the University.* It began at 10 p.m. and it went on until 4 a.m. with a slight remission at 2 o'clock. We had 1,000 tons of petrol in the garage and nothing would have been found if we had been hit. Hitherto I had been wont to

---

* The Good Friday Blitz took place on April 11, 1941. Winston Churchill visited the next day, April 12.

walk round without my tin hat, since a bomb would give me an honorable discharge from a life which seemed to have nothing to offer. This night, because of G.'s genuine distress, I put one on.

An H.E.* descended on to John Wright's printing works on the Center not a hundred yards away. As we wandered out of the door to see what had happened, a shower of papers came down, sheets of books, like a pamphlet raid all over the town. Behind Wright's was a narrow little lane called Christmas Street, one of the oldest parts of Bristol with houses made chiefly of wood leaning towards each other from age. One directly abutting the printing works had already caught fire and it would not be long before the flames spread across the narrow street. A little house just opposite the boss had a store of tires in the upstairs room, for I had been sent to take an inventory of them a week before, and tires at that time were in very short supply.

That wave of bombers had passed so we could safely leave the garage for a few minutes. We ran up the street and I leapt up the stairs and rolled tires down them to G. at the bottom who sent them on their way down the sloping lane with a shove. Big tires and small tires bounced down. They were all brand new. Then the flames began licking at the stairs and G. called me down. We collected all those which had stopped on the way and piled them outside the fish and chip shop on the corner. A special constable then stopped us from going back to see if there was anything more we could do. It was just as well. In ten minutes time a second H.E. which had fallen into John Wright's all unknown, went off and the roof of the house flew up into the air and tires we had left went sailing out of the windows in all directions.

We rolled our stock back to the garage and waited till morning to receive the boss's congratulations and in hopes of the customary monetary reward that firms were wont to give firewatchers for saving their property. The former we received rather perfunctorily, of the latter we saw nothing. It seemed the boss would rather have gathered in the insurance money for the whole stock. And that day the fish and chip shop was closed and a notice outside read: "Danger. Unexploded Bomb Under Counter."

Only one other blitz was memorable. It was not a real one and came after the "season" was over. We were asleep one night on the floor when a

* HE likely stands for "high explosive." During World War II, high-explosive bombs were dropped by both German and Allied forces. Sometimes they did not explode right away. Indeed, some have stayed in place for decades and remain both live and extremely dangerous.

distant thud awoke me. It was followed by another louder and then a third thud which shook the place slightly. I thumped G. who was always a powerful sleeper and rolled under the table. A terrific crash came just behind us and the floor shook. G. opened one eye and said sleepily: "Is there a blitz or something?" Before I could tell him what I thought of him there was another crash in front of us and this time a shower of glass and bricks fell all around us as G., awake at last dived under the table with me. No more followed.

It turned out to be a wounded German plane going home which had decided to unload its last stick over Bristol. The last but one crash behind us had fallen on the Eye Hospital and the last of all on a store just across the road, shattering it and our plate glass windows, which had been replaced after the first blitz. The road was a sea of glass and it was the only road through the middle of the town. We fetched the wide garage brooms and swept it clear at two o'clock in the morning. Next day we were to hear that the local police had commended our action to the boss.

During the blitzes and with G. for a friend I was relatively happy. When the time came for him to leave the outlook was dark indeed. He went in the autumn and the next Boxing Day he came to see me in his bell bottoms and secreting something inside his coat. He had come up from Plymouth by train on house leave and, knowing that I would have had no Christmas dinner he had risked "jankers" to steal a bit of turkey for me from the mess.* But his train had been delayed and on the way for many hours and being hungry he had eaten a nibble every now and then. Rather shamefacedly he produced what was left, a wing bone wrapped round in its skin. Deeply touched, nevertheless, I devoured the skin and sucked the bone. It had the taste of turkey anyway!

Nearly a year went by and then the first step was taken—although it did not seem so at the time. Overworked I was given a weekend off in the summer and went to Weston-super-Mare for a rest. Accommodation was scarce and I got a room but no food. For some time past I had had odd dizzy spells and [whenever I felt one coming on] at once instinct had driven me to look for food even if I did not feel hungry. Having eaten I felt all right again. That afternoon I walked along the promenade and as I looked at the beach black with people I wondered idly what would happen if there was one of the newly-started Baedeker raids on

---

* "Jankers" is a British military term for Restriction of Privileges—a minor infraction.

Weston.* Exeter had already suffered. Next morning I went out in search of breakfast and awoke some hours later in the local hospital. It was the first of what was to be a series of hypoglycemic attacks, due to a sudden drop in the blood sugar level.

I had fallen forward striking the ground full force with my forehead, and was a shocking mess. My face was swollen, blue and green and with a graze all down my nose and mouth. I was a sight indeed! By this time I was wearing sports coat and flannels, when not in overalls and was shaving twice weekly. The house surgeon asked me my name and when I told him he said I was still wandering in my mind from concussion. Wearily I handed them my identity card, luckily one of the green ones with [a] photograph, a useful relic of my few F.A.N.Y. days. I was put to bed in a men's ward, nevertheless, and that night came the first Baedeker blitz on Weston which I had anticipated.† I lay there quite detached from my surroundings and watched through the windows the flashes of various hues, parachute flairs, incendiaries, and tracer bullets chasing each other across the sky. I felt as if I were a being from another world, quite unconnected with this carnage.

The ward filled rapidly and next morning we were all packed into ambulances and taken off to Bath where a Nissen Hut Hospital had been erected at Coombe Down. There I stayed five weeks. Just before I left it was found I also had had a scaphoid fracture of my left wrist and my arm was put into plaster. There was no question of convalescence for I had nowhere to go, so back to the garage, shaky and weak to pick up the threads of work and firewatching.

Six months later I passed out again in the street and was taken to the British Royal Infirmary with a cut head. Here I remained two weeks and this was to be the beginning of my emancipation. There was a kindly house surgeon of [a] well-known Quaker family from Bath and when he had heard my story and examined me he brought along a plastic surgeon to see me. In addition a blood sugar test was done which not only proved conclusively that my blackouts were due to hypoglycemia, but very nearly killed me.

The plastic surgeon said he would remove the small but persistent breast tissue and would then put me in touch with a bigger plastic surgeon

---

* The Baedeker raids were a retaliatory pattern of bombing taken up by the Germans and the British beginning in March 1942. Rather than targeting strategic military or governmental sites, these raids aimed for popular cultural or historical sites, places that might be recommended in so-called Baedeker guidebooks. They chipped away profoundly at morale.

† The raid on Weston-super-Mare took place on June 27, 1942.

to whom he had himself been student. And why not get re-registered, he asked?

It was as if a sudden tiny gleam of light had appeared showing a possible line of escape from what had been a prison of darkness. Whichever way I had turned I had seemed to be hemmed in by birth certificates, identity cards, driving licenses and my mail as it was addressed to me. If I tried to change my job or if I were to start in a new town, it would be the same. Everyone would know at once and everyone would tell everyone else. Re-registration? Was it possible?

I returned to the garage when my scalp wound had healed with the promise of a bed in the surgeon's hospital whenever there was one available. It would not be difficult to get leave from the boss since my black outs could be given as the cause. At least there seemed to be some hope.

On the morning of the very day I was due to be admitted for surgery I had another blackout and once again woke up in the casualty department of the Infirmary. They were becoming used to it by now. That afternoon the good house surgeon had me transferred to the other hospital and, in consultation with the surgeon they suggested it might be as well to do a laparotomy to see if there was any tumor of the pancreas which could produce such virulent hypoglycemic reactions, these being due to sudden output of insulin into the blood. But what was causing this output?

The chest operation was carried out first and pentothal and cyclopropane was used to put me to sleep. When I came round I vomited for twenty four hours, to the annoyance of all concerned who had assured me that no one ever vomited after these modern anesthetics, which were not like the old ether which I had had for my tonsils when a child. But this was to be the pattern for all operations. It seemed I took anesthetics very badly, becoming violent after going under and coming back from the theater with bruises on arms and legs where I had been held down by tough orderlies, and always vomiting and vomiting. But that was not till later.

I was delighted with this operation when I had recovered from it. At last I was rid of what I hated most. I sat out on the verandah letting the sun help to heal the incisions. Then ten days later I went up to the theater for the abdominal examination.

Anyone who has had a long slit down their abdomen and then spent the night vomiting alone can imagine what it was like. Moreover the operation was abortive. There was nothing to be found but to give me my money's worth they took out my appendix for luck, as it were. Oddly enough no one seemed to have thought of carrying the examination further to see what was abnormal otherwise.

I had made friends with another firewatcher who lived with his sister in a flat and having heard I was in hospital he offered to let me convalesce for five days at his place and his sister would look after me. It was much appreciated for two operations had taken their toll but when the five days were up I was back in the office firewatching and working, though lightly at first, by day. I also had the information on how to become re-registered as a male and acquire new Christian names.

I had become acquainted some months before with a doctor in Bath who was prepared to sign a medical certificate, and then I needed one from a member of my family. This would be impossible from the aunts or my brother. I wrote therefore to a cousin whom I knew but little but who was more modern than anyone else. She was the daughter of Auntie Grace of Worthing and so my first cousin although it was her son who was really my contemporary. Having for some time suspected something she readily obliged to my delight, for I had met her hardly half a dozen times in my life. And Somerset House accepted the application and I became Laurence Michael, at last. This was the year following the operation, 1943.*

Now it would be necessary to inform the aunts and to have a change made in the form of address of correspondents. Toto, Daisy and Maudie, had, contrary to all expectation, when Folkestone was evacuated after Dunkirk, gone to stay at Mrs. Hearne's hotel in Hertfordshire. Once or twice I had visited them there for a day or so, and had met a friend of theirs who was a lady doctor, whom I liked and thought it would be best if she broke the news as gently as possible since they would believe her as being a doctor whereas they would not believe anyone else.

Toto's reaction was that God made them male and female, she had never heard of His making them intersex as well.† Daisy said she had never heard

---

* Liz Hodgkinson's *Michael née Laura* includes an image of the "certified copy of an entry of birth" that shows the reregistration occurring on April 14, 1944. Dillon/Jivaka's text is ambiguous. Does "this was the year following the operation, 1943" mean that the operation was in 1943 and the application was accepted in 1944, or that the chest surgery occurred in 1942 and the application was accepted in 1943?

† Here Dillon/Jivaka uses the term "intersex" in much the way it is still used, namely, to indicate ambiguity of biological sex. Dillon had previously discussed the topic in his book *Self: A Study in Ethics and Endocrinology* (London: Heinemann Medical Books, 1946), there mainly using the (now outdated and pejorative) term "hermaphrodite" (particularly in Chapter 4, 57–74). As reflected in quotations from several news accounts from May 1958, disclosing his transition,

of it either but if it could happen then I would be the most likely person it could happen to, and Maudie merely snorted. But the hurdle was now past.

With the poker-face back on and on the defensive I went to get a new identity card at the Labor Exchange, prepared for grins and curiosity. "Oh, yes," said the man behind the counter, "we have had quite a lot of these applications," and made me out a new card without batting an eyelid! How common was it? I am none the wiser on that point now.*

Then I automatically received my call-up papers for the Army although I was told that the medical examination would be a mere formality. "Yes," said the Army doctor, "we've turned down a lot like you."

So back to the garage I went where everyone knew and things were no better in consequence. But this good lady doctor had put a suggestion to me: why not take a medical degree? And persistently she had written the same theme again and again. But I did not want to, having no desire to be a doctor. Then after re-registration it occurred to me it might be a way out, especially if I could start in a university where I was not known, and I was intended in research on the relation of mind and body. But I had done no science at school and for six years I had learned nothing and read only for amusement. Physics, chemistry, zoology and botany were required as a Pre-medical examination.

With permission from the boss now that the best part of the war was over, I joined the Merchant Venturers' Technical College, going for lectures and practical work in these subjects in the mornings and working with the cars for the rest of the day. It was the first time that I was able to start among people who knew nothing whatever about me and accepted me as an ordinary young man. The relief was indescribable.

Meanwhile I had had a day off and been to Basingstoke to interview Sir Harold Gillies, the word's leading plastic surgeon, to whom the Bristol surgeon had recommended me. He had examined me from all angles and asked many questions. Then he gave his verdict:

"I think your case merits surgical interference. I will put you down as an acute hypospadic."

---

he seemed to view himself as likely intersex. Whether he was aware of the term transsexual (first used by David Cauldwell in 1949) or not, Dillon/Jivaka never used trans- terminology of any sort to refer to himself.

* In *But for the Grace: The True Story of a Dual Existence* (London: W. H. Allen & Co., 1954), Robert Allen (who like Dillon had been assigned female at birth) explains that his reregistration took place on October 30, 1944.

The world began to seem worth living in after all. Not even his added regrets that he could not start yet because, since the landings in France had just begun, his hands were full with returning casualties, discouraged me somewhat. Indeed at this time he was operating from eight in the morning until four the next morning and this certainly contributed to his later vascular trouble.

I was prepared to wait. To wait with hope in one's heart is easy. And I had waited long enough without any. So back I went to study science and to park cars.

But there was still another problem that had to be dealt with. If I went to a University I would need to show evidence of my Oxford M.A. and the certificate was in the wrong name. I wrote to Jimmy McKie who was then a Major in the Army Intelligence and on the verge of sailing for Germany. This was not his first intimation of things. I had broken the news of my change over to him earlier and I had met him for a day in Oxford in my new clothes. But his wife who was a sergeant in the N.A.A.F. and stationed at Hendon, did not yet know.* I left it to him to tell her when my registration was completed.

It was due to the kindness and commonsense of my ex-tutor that my name was transferred to the books of Brasenose College where I had learned all my philosophy, and also that the Oxford University Registrar was persuaded to issue me an M.A. certificate with only my initials in place of my first names. Jimmy McKie then composed a masterpiece of a reference, which did not use any pronoun whatsoever and yet was perfectly grammatical and readable. But then words were always his hobby as those who knew him will know.

Now to find a suitable University! All were crowded out with ex-servicemen who had taken war-time degrees or had their courses interrupted, and my lack of the first Pre-medical Examination hindered me. I sat for Edinburgh and failed. I sat for London First M.B. and failed. My six years of non-learning now made memorizing very difficult. Then I tried Trinity College, Dublin, which has affiliations with Oxford and Cambridge and interchangeable degrees and after an interview I was accepted for their Pre-medical year to learn those four subjects on the groundwork of what I had picked up at the Merchant Venturers.

But what about Bobby? He lived but 26 miles from Dublin and would be very angry if his name was linked with mine since I was such a freak and

---

* NAAF stood for Northwest African Air Forces, which during 1943 formed part of the Allied Mediterranean Air Command.

had done the most outrageous thing in changing over. He was desperately self-conscious about having me for a sister and he would never own me as a brother. And he did not. We met, after about seven years apart and had lunch together in the restaurant of the Savoy cinema. He accepted the fact of my residence in Dublin as a *fait accompli* that could not be altered, but begged me never to couple my name with his or to admit to any relationship. Nor might I visit him at his home. Seeing how genuinely embarrassed he was I agreed to all this for I no more wanted any publicity than he did, although we might safely have assumed a cousin relationship I thought, but he did not agree.

My interviews both with the University and my brother finished, I returned to England for the summer. In 1939 I had begun to write a small book, popular scientific on the subject of intersex from the point of view of the physical as well as the psychological and moral. It had been finished during those evenings at the garage when the blitzes were over and now I set about finding a publisher for it, successfully at the second attempt. The last chapter had been entitled "Free Will" and was purely philosophical. Therein I had suggested that the usual way of looking at the problem of pre-determination was back to front. If one can answer the question "Could I have done otherwise?" in the affirmative then one has not acted freely since one can only have acted with a part of one's self, following a desire or an emotion or a particular reason. If the answer was in the negative then one had acted freely since one had acted with the whole of oneself and no part had been left out which could afterwards regret the action. Many years later I was to find this consonant with Mahayana philosophy but at that time I felt I was on the threshold of Truth; stretching out my hands towards it into a completely dark room. It was there but I could not see it.

Next the Bath doctor who had been ill asked me to drive him to his Scottish home and to stay a week to see if I could help with his son, also a doctor who had had a nervous breakdown and was in a paranoiac state and refused to do any work but spent all day bemoaning his fate.

This led to an odd experience. The doctor was married with a wife and two young girl children ages eight and five. They were staying in a house in a nearby town while he was with his parents in the country a few miles away. After I had been there a few days he suddenly decided to go and stay with his family and made me promise to come and spend each day with him. On the afternoon of my second day visiting him he was walking with me to the bus stop to see me off back to his parents' house when he began begging me not to go but to stay the night with him. I told him his father expected me back and that I had nothing with me for the night but the nearer we came to the stop the more insistent he became. Finally I capitulated and we walked back to the house.

After supper he began his usual arguments about the state of the world and the badness of everybody but on this occasion as I began to argue back as usual, the feeling came upon me that I was becoming involved in a tremendous struggle with some Force of Evil. On and on it went and I held on knowing that I must not give up the fight, unaware of the nature of my adversary, and externally we were just arguing as usual. At eleven o'clock at night suddenly it all fell away and I knew I had won the battle. The arguments also ceased and I fell exhausted on the settee utterly, utterly tired out but thankful that I had been the victor.

What was it all about? I had not the slightest idea. It was just a matter of feeling. Next day I asked him why he had so persisted in having me stay that night but he refused to tell me then, saying only that he would tell me some other time. I left the next day to return to Bristol and saw him about a month later and again I asked him "Why did you insist on my staying that night?" His reply shook me badly. He said:

"Because I made up my mind to kill my wife and children and then commit suicide. The world is not a fit place to bring children into and they would have been better out of it. If you hadn't stayed I would have done so."

So that was the Force of Evil I had been aware of yet could not identify. Apparently some better or saner part of him had held him back on the proviso that I stayed to help him.

There were two things the aunts had always taught me to have nothing to do with, Roman Catholicism, especially Jesuits, and the Occult, and indeed I had never been interested in either. The latter seemed half false and half dangerous, and previously I had had no contact with anything concerning it. But this young half-mad doctor had dabbled in it, so he told me, though to what extent and in what way I do not know. I did not want to know. Whether false or not it was certainly dangerous from the effect it could have on the susceptible mind.

But one more thing happened this summer, the one thing of supreme importance. I had my first plastic surgery operation, and I made the acquaintance of famous Rooksdown House near Basingstoke, where officers and men and women of the Army and Navy and from civil raid or accidents were being given new faces, new hands, and new hope. It was to be the first of thirteen operations before I was completed and they were spread over the next four years. In term time I was the medical student in Dublin, on the last day of term I would fly to London and be at Rooksdown by midnight, often to have an operation the very next morning, and back again on the last day of the vacation bandaged and in need of daily dressings for a week or more. Thus I came to know hospital life from the patient's point of view as well as the doctor's, an advantage which many of my colleagues lacked, and lacking were unaware how genuine were the complaints from the bed very often with which they lacked the sympathy that experience would have given them.

PART II

Conquest of the Mind

CHAPTER 6

Medical Student

How different was life now! I could walk past anyone and not fear to hear any comments for no one looked at me twice. Of course the fact that I was twelve years older than any of my fellow students made the lack of any real companionship still felt, and junior students did not hobnob with the Registrars who were of nearer age to me. But the elderly Professor of Zoology, an old Oxford man himself, became a good friend and invited me down to stay with him sometimes at his cottage in Arklow. It was his eldest son who was then house-surgeon at the Royal City of Dublin hospital, in whom I confided, since someone had to do my dressings for me. And he was faithful to his trust and when the time came for him to leave he passed me on to the surgical registrar who was also staunch and never revealed to any colleague what he knew. He happened to be a friend of Bobby and was intrigued to discover what had happened to the sister Bob was known to have had, who had not been seen since childhood, but he never told even Bobby that he knew. Would that all could be so faithful to a confidence!

I passed the Pre-Medical examination though hardly with flying colors. My Oxford training had left me with the tendency to discuss a question rather than to answer as per the textbook and only in Zoology did I do well, since the Professor understood that type of mentality which Oxford produces. But the worst hurdle was to be Anatomy, for it was sheer learning by heart and when a brain has lain idle for six years it does not take kindly to memorizing again, whereas my fellow students, only just out of school, had not lost the art.

Naturally the temptation to join the Boat Club and pick up the threads of rowing was very great. I was now 11 stone and well developed muscularly from garage work.* The scars on my chest might be difficult to explain but I had decided to attribute everything, including the need for operations during vacations, to blitz damage and since blitzes were an unknown quantity to the Southern Irish, no one could say definitely that they might not have been the cause. But there was a further problem, less easily solved. Oxford rowed the orthodox style while Trinity favored a rather spurious type of Fairbairnism. Rowing men will know that the gulf between the bigoted adherents of each style is as rigid as that between Roman Catholic and Protestant. If I rowed it would have to be Fairbairn which was anathema to me.

Yet so great was the urge to handle an oar once more that I decided to adapt myself, and at the first summer's regatta I rowed No. 2 in the Second Eight, being awarded my Junior Eight Colors. But my particular brand of humor demanded that after my Oxford "blue" I would be satisfied with nothing less than Senior Eight Colors. Of course they knew nothing of the facts of my rowing antecedents, as I claimed the Brasenose Second Eight in lieu of the truth. So in the Hilary term of my fourth year I stroked the First Eight after an unexpected win in a scratch crew against three other crews in an unofficial regatta always held at the end of the Christmas term. Contrary to all expectation we had beaten the Senior Eight in a race which had immediately followed upon a close fight with a crew made up of old oarsmen. So furious were we at being made to race again without a rest that we ended two lengths ahead of our astonished and ashamed Senior Eight, although we were composed only of a mixture of second and third eight men. I was stroking and my sense of justice had been upset. For Trinity standards and those of Oxford were different in many respects as I was to find: training rules were not kept rigidly and coxing in Ireland as a whole was dirty in the extreme, since the aim was to win at all costs, rather than to win fairly.

Next term I stroked the Senior Eight in the annual event against Belfast but it was then discovered that I would not be eligible for the Ladies' Plate

* Eleven stone is 154 pounds.

at Henley, since an Edwardian rule forbade any oarsman who had been matriculated more than five years from taking part. This was because, in those palmy days, young men addicted to sport and not a whit to study, would remain undergraduates for many years, and the Ladies' Plate is specifically an undergraduate affair, not open to town clubs or regular oarsmen.

So that summer I was given a four to stroke at the annual Trinity regatta to allow me to receive my Senior Eight Colors but if I could not go to Henley I could not row in the Senior Eight any more, for this was the peak of the rowing endeavor each year. Next year, therefore, I joined the Neptune Boat Club, a town club, and viewed the College regattas through the eyes of the town boys who regarded the undergraduates as "snooty" in the extreme.

It may be wondered how I could row after having so many operations, for every vacation for my first four years was spent in hospital. On the evening of the last day of term I would fly over to London and take the train to Basingstoke, arriving at midnight and as often as not my operation would have been scheduled for the morning. But skin grafting did not involve muscle cutting and though I once went out on rowing practice with 8 stitches in me, it did no harm.

But on my fifth visit things went wrong. Always addicted to hematomas, that bugbear of every surgeon, due to [an] unduly slow clotting time of the blood, the operation, which was one of crucial importance, broke down and infection set in, so that I was unable to return for the Hilary term and spent three months in hospital, and when I emerged for the summer term, my upper legs had been denuded of their top layer of skin for replacement grafts and more hematoma had appeared even on these graft areas, so that they looked as if strawberry jam had been spread over them. I walked with a stick and felt far from well.

I failed the Anatomy examination at my first attempt, less because of this than because it entailed sheer memory work and the six years of the war had left me quite out of practice in learning and my brain seemed to be against getting into practice again. At the second attempt I managed to scrape through with just over the fifty percent required.

The student having to go into hospital idly thinks what a wonderful, quiet place it will be to work in and how he will have nothing to do all day but study. How quickly is he disillusioned! After an operation or during an illness one seems to lack the mental energy required for anything more serious than a thriller or funny story or the daily newspaper.

Not that Rooksdown House was in the least typical of a hospital. Sir Harold had refused to have it so. Patients with badly burned faces and bodies might have to keep on coming back as stage by stage the damage was repaired, and some had had as many as sixty operations. If there was strict hospital discipline, he felt that many would give up returning and go away half finished; and to Sir Harold the making of life normal again for those who were mutilated, whether by man or by Nature, was all-important. It was to this he devoted his own life and it was to this that I owed mine.

The first thing that any patient learned who was brought in was to stop feeling sorry for himself. There was always someone in another bed who was worse than he. And so those who knew they were disfigured took courage again. The second thing we learned was never to help anyone if he could possibly do it for himself, especially those with hand injuries who must be made to use their fingers at all costs. Naturally people were ready to assist when it was obvious assistance was necessary but otherwise men learned to feed with one hand without having to have their food cut up for them, to dress and even to make their beds. It was all part of the healing scheme.

We felt that Rooksdown was more of a country club than anything else. When we returned we would greet old friends and be introduced to new ones. Often the same ones would be back again or due back and their arrival would be eagerly awaited. On the morning of an operation the patient would be much ragged over his missing breakfast and would be given a hearty send-off to the theater. Despite the pain of awakening we were light-hearted about it all and this was wholly due to Sir Harold's policy.

Some of the friends I made there merit mention. There was the Fleet Air Arm Lieutenant who, according to textbook teaching should have been dead, for he had had more than one third of his body burned. Returning to his carrier on fire he had ditched the burning plane deliberately in the sea so that he should not endanger the ship. His whole face was burned, both ears gone, the ends of all his fingers and his arms to above the elbow and his legs from below the knees. Only where his shorts and shirt had saved him a little was he free.

Slowly they made parts, nose, chin, ears, gave him an artificial eye and taught him to use the stumps of his fingers. His fiancée stuck close to him and in the end married him despite that he said his face looked like the back of a bus after a smash, and he took up the teaching career he had left and became justly the hero of the boy's school where he worked.

Another one wore his navel under his armpit. He had been burnt all down one side of face and chest and the axilla was badly damaged. This had been due to a stove busting in a hut in France when he was cooking himself some supper. It was interesting to learn that a few more of the war-time casualties were due to accidents, than to enemy action. They had raised tube-pedicles crucifers from the flesh of his abdomen and swung them up until the skin could be spread and the axilla covered, and the wound was in the middle! These tube pedicles were Sir Harold's own invention and by their means flesh from one part of the body could be used to cover a distant part, but each movement required a separate operation and time for healing.

Then there was the factory girl who, unmindful of instructions about wearing a cap, had had her long hair caught in a machine and her whole scalp torn off. No Red Indian could have done the job better. Skin from her back was slowly transferred and when the skull was covered a wig solved the problem.

A young engineer petty officer in the Royal Navy had been standing too near the machinery one day and as the ship listed his overalls and his private parts were caught and torn off. The nature of his operations was similar to my own. But when he went on leave and told the father of the girl he had been engaged to, in honorable fashion what had happened, he was driven from the house and told never to come near the daughter again.

The beauty of Basingstoke was that the inhabitants quickly became accustomed to seeing the Rooksdown patients about the town with appalling scarring or strange pieces of flesh attached to them as pedicles were joined, and they ceased to look twice at us. This gave those conscious of their facial injuries confidence to go out but, they said, when they went on leave, as soon as the train reached the next station their troubles began. Then people would stare or look pitying or hastily look the other way in repulsion. While the war was on there was sympathy but not long after it was over people began to let their aversion become apparent—so I was told by one Rooksdown friend I met by chance in the streets of Dublin. He had had a burned face and a new nose made, so excellently that no one would have known. But his mouth had contracted and he had to have it enlarged since he could not force an ordinary dessert spoon in, and for this a pedicle had been raised and joined to his chin.

They were not without their sense of humor either. One fellow had lost both ears [but] the surgeon concentrated [first] on his nose. But after one leave he came back and begged to have his ears done first. The plastic pair had to be stuck on with a special glue and removed on going to bed and he said, "When the chambermaid in my hotel came in, in the morning with my jug of hot water and saw my ears lying on the washing stand . . ." The rest was always lost in a great roar of laughter whenever he told the story.

In the early stages the surgeons had not discovered that a hairy part transplanted grows its hair with equal facility anywhere it may be put. Thus one man had a tuft growing on the end of his thumb and another developed a hairy nose, before it was noted.

Rooksdown men formed a club primarily to help those members who were in need as the result of their injuries and anyone who had had a plastic operation done there was eligible to join. We wore badges of a rook and there was an annual "old boy's day" in the summer with a garden party when we would meet old friends now long finished.

At Christmas, too, there was a grand party on the Eve, which I M.C.'d twice from a wheelchair, thus making my debut into the social world from which I had been so long debarred. There were games and dancing for those able and a huge supper. Then in the morning the Sister and nurses would have breakfast with us and at lunch Sir Harold would be deputed to carve the turkey. It was to be expected he would do so with professional skill. But no! A human body, yes, he was a sculptor in human flesh no less, but when it came to a turkey . . . The turkey ended up on the floor and the ward sister had to take over the knife!

But alas, when Sir Harold became ill and had to retire for awhile with Buerger's disease (the same as what the king had), the plastic surgeon who deputized for him, thought to improve on the country club atmosphere and tried to turn the place into a hospital. In this he was aided by a new matron who objected to patients going off to the cinema without special permission or to seeing a man with a patch over one eye, riding a bicycle down the corridor at ten o'clock at night! And finally she forbade the nurses to breakfast with us on Christmas morning and nearly produced a rebellion.

Back and forth, back and forth I flew. Patient and budding doctor alternately. Then came the day when I had passed all the preliminary examinations and started work in the hospital, that same Royal City of Dublin where I had been to have my wounds dressed so often.

The Dublin hospitals are roughly divided into those for Protestants and those for Catholics with a couple who have a mixture, although in no case was there complete exclusion of the other religionists. But religion is the pivot of Irish life and the dispute between the two sects is irreconcilable and often violent.

Mine was a Protestant hospital, but naturally the patients and nurses were mainly Catholic, while the medical staff was mainly Protestant. On my very first day, arriving a term late because of being put back by failing Anatomy, I found myself in a clinic with the senior of all the clinicians, old "Alfie" Parsons, as he was called, reputed to be eighty or more. He was invaluable in that, belonging to the old school, he made sure we knew something of the history of various discoveries and also he liked to teach the classical origins of various terms. In this I scored heavily, because, knowing Greek I could derive most terms even if I did not actually know what they should mean.

Seeing a new face among the students beside the bed he was clinicing on, he said "Doctor, what's athetosis?" He always called us "Doctor" in ironical anticipation. The woman patient in the bed was waving her hand about in odd fashion trying to reach something and unable to. The derivation of athetosis was un-placing. "Not being able to place," I said, then added, looking at the woman—"your hands where you want to." Dr. Parsons was just turning away to attack another victim when he spun round on his heel.

"Are you a classical scholar, doctor?" He demanded to know.

"Well, I suppose so, sir, sort of," I said most embarrassed. Thereafter he invariably asked me for derivations of terms in his clinics only some of which I knew.

Although eighty he was so energetic we were often hard put to keep up with him when we were on as his clinical clerks. Each student had to do one month with each honorary, learning how to take histories, for he would be the first to interview the new patient, then he would have to tell the house surgeon or house physician what he had found. Next morning he would have to answer an intensive questioning on the case from "his man."

In Dublin we did not refer to the honoraries as "chief" as seems to be done in English hospitals. They were always "my man" or in the commonly heard Northern Ireland accent, "M' marn." "Y'r marn's up the house" would be the way of informing a fellow student that his honorary had come in unseen, and then the missing student would fly from the common room up the stairs, and there were four flights of them, asking every one he met: "Where's m' marn?" and eventually arrive breathless at the bedside where "the marn" was already examining the patient and would be wanting to know whether it was your custom to sleep at such an hour, or he might merely drop the cliché "better late than never, I suppose."

The most valuable thing about our whole medical course was the time students had to do in residence in the hospital, unlike their English fellows. The minimum was two months, the maximum what you would. You paid for the privilege of doing all the dog work and so gaining invaluable experience. Each month you would change "your man," and when you were surgical dresser, as it was called, you assisted in the theater, a thing that no unqualified student elsewhere seems to be allowed to do. If you were very lucky, before you had passed your Finals you might even be allowed to do an operation, under the eagle eye of the surgeon, of course, and in my last term as a student I did my first appendectomy thus, quite successfully.

If you were on with a physician you had to do an early morning round of the patients and test all the urines left with test tubes in a rack on a table in the wards. Immediately after breakfast clinics began. If "your man" was clinicing you had to have a blackboard and easel in the ward and the bed pulled out into the middle and the whole case at your fingertips. But you would only be called on to answer when the other students had been given their turn. These would come from any of the Dublin hospitals, since it was the reputation of the man clinicing which counted, and some popular clinicians would have as many as eighty students crammed into a ward or trying to listen from the corridor. And, of course, as Finals drew near the orders of future examiners would be especially full, in hopes of picking up a hint of their favorite topics which might give a clue to a future question.

But those who were in residence also had to work a rota in the Accident Department and whoever's turn it was to be on had a twenty-four hour shift to do. Every accident, however trite, which came in he had to see first and attend to if he could, stitching wounds, sounding chests or advising on babies' diarrhea. If it was too big for him to handle he would call the house-man on duty and if it was still too big the surgeon or physician would be summoned by telephone. If an emergency operation was needed it would not be the surgical dresser but the resident student on duty who would as-sist, first preparing the patient, shaving the area, testing urine and blood pressure and notifying the theater. Thus the clinical clerks might still have theater experience on their months with a physician, if they were on Acci-dent duty. By this means we saw a great deal more cases than anyone could see merely attending a few hours during the day. Unfortunately when the scheme for making housemanship compulsory for one year, before final qualification, came into force, the resident student could no longer be ad-mitted, and the loss must have been great for those who followed shortly after us.

On Friday and Saturday nights the ambulance would bring in an assort-ment of drunks with various head injuries whom they had picked up off the streets after they had consumed their weeks pay. We even had a "drunk room," a closet in the Accident Department, where drunks could sleep off the effects of their excesses. But what we resented most was being woken up for a toothache, which could have gone to the dentist and had not, or the extracted tooth that continued to bleed or the pain that "I've had for days, doctor." For we went to bed hopeful of a quiet night always.

Once I fell foul of my colleagues, two Belfast men and one Australian student, because they would come to bed at one in the morning and not put any restraint on the noise they made, shouting or singing as if it were day. In the fracas that followed I had my left elbow momentarily dislocated and the ulna nerve torn which necessitated two operations by "my marn" and added to the toll of Rooksdown with which I had not yet finished and also put an end to my rowing for that year. For the torn nerve had to be put round to the front of the elbow to prevent its being continually irritated by anything touching it as it hung loose instead of being in its groove, and even now the elbow will not straighten completely. Doubtless had I been a young student with a father to make a row, notice might have been taken of it, but as it was, the delinquents, who had been three to my one, got off with a reprimand, the hospital not wanting any publicity about the matter.

In our fifth year we had to go to the Rotunda for our midwifery month. Strangely reluctant to go in, I was equally reluctant to leave when my time was up. We first had to see two cases in the labor room and then we were on "district" in groups of four, two who had done a fortnight and two new ones. If it "moved fast," as the saying was, our turn would be round again within a day or two. If slow, we, near the top of the list, might have to stay on the premises for days on end awaiting a case. If the baby was an easy delivery we did it ourselves. If it was a breech or had any complications, or there was abnormal bleeding one of us would go back to fetch the Clinical Clerk who was qualified and doing his D.G.O. and he would come out in the van. If it was beyond his powers he would send the ambulance to take the mother into hospital. Thus was the whole district served. No one, however poor, if she had registered ante-natally, need fear being without medical assistance at the time of labor, and she should have reported monthly to the out-patients department for check-ups. If any trouble was anticipated the patient would be admitted when labor began. According to her means she would pay for her maintenance, but all treatment was free. Yet when the demand for national health began, lies were freely told about mothers being left to die for want of money to take them to hospital.* Only those who refused to attend had their babies by themselves.

A grubby small boy or his anxious father would arrive and hand an equally grubby bit of paper to the porter who would call the group on

* Dillon was in medical school amid intense debate about, and the new implementation of, socialized medicine in various parts of the United Kingdom. England's National Health Service Act passed in 1946.

duty and out we would go with our little bags of instruments, at any hour of day or night. The house would very likely be one of the slum tenements of Dublin which used to be a fine Georgian residence and now each great room was the home of one family, and the windows were blocked up with plywood or paper, the broad staircase filthy and paintless, the paper hanging off the walls, and behind the strips bugs and lice.

The patient would be lying on a dirty bed covered with newspapers and with a blanket of sorts over her. Once I sat down on the bed and a squeal and a wriggle informed me I had all but sat on a three year old urchin who crawled out from beside his mother indignantly and was driven out of the room. There would be the midwife also present; a greasy fat old woman from upstairs or next door with strands of hair hanging down over her face who would respectfully leave when the doctors arrived. While we made our examination of the patient someone would be boiling a kettle to make us tea, which they regarded as an essential to our work or their own ideas of hospitality, and we would have to force ourselves to drink the black brew from dirty, cracked cups. Then we would sit down and wait for things to happen, sometimes dozing or perhaps playing cards. We quickly found out that so long as the woman on the bed only screamed "Jesus" or "Holy Mary!" the time had not yet come. When she let out a shrill "Jesus, Mary, Joseph!" all three, then we must be up and doing for then the baby was really on its way. It was an infallible guide to the progress of labor!

Then one of the group had to visit the case daily for the next ten days or it would be docked from our requisite number of twenty which must be done in the month to count for the course. On one Sunday morning I was on my way by motorcycle, a new Royal Enfield, to a new housing estate, when a dog belonging to a newspaper seller ran out barking at the cycle. I kicked at it but instead of running away it gripped my leg with its teeth and with difficulty I shook it off while the bike veered across the fortunately empty road and ended up outside a doctor's house. A crowd quickly gathered as I examined the injury. The skin had not been broken but it had torn a vein inside the muscle and one of my familiar hematomas was developing with rapid swelling. Everyone pointed to the brass plate on the door so I went in and had first aid done by the doctor who ran me back to the Rotunda in his car allowing me to leave my bike in his garden. In the excitement of all this and being temporarily crippled, I forgot to tell anyone I had not reached the patient, and the case was docked from our group to our immense indignation at such injustice, since I had been on my way to it at the time. However there was no remedy, but to do another one to make up the total.

The month at the Rotunda finished, I returned to my hospital for daily clinics, no longer the shy student I had been but knowing the ways of the clinicians and chuckling at the discomfort of the new students as we had been chuckled at ourselves when we were new. Some time after I had qualified I read in some English newspaper of a campaign to preserve the ego of the medical student more. It complained that there was too much twisting of the students' tails by the clinicing doctors so that they were embarrassed at being made fools of or reproved in front of a ward full of patients.

In our early days we did feel embarrassed but we also remembered the details for which we had suffered embarrassment and so were less likely to make the same mistake twice. And a mistake may cost a patient his life. In recent years man has become very sensitive about his ego and the more it is cosseted the more undisciplined and egoistic does he become.

Dr. "Alfie" Parsons was a past master of the art of tail-twisting. To a brand new class he asked the question, "What is the normal body temperature, doctor?" "98.4," replied the man he had tapped on the chest with his stethoscope. "And what do you think it is?" he swung round on a girl student of which there were many. Since 98.4 had apparently found no favor, she tried "98.6, sir." He turned on his heel and went out of the room. One student braver than the rest ran after him.

"Excuse me, sir," he said, "but what is the normal temperature?" Dr. Parsons looked him up and down.

"I never heard it was anything but 98.4, doctor," he said witheringly.

Sometimes it was the patients who caused amusement. The senior surgeon was clinicing on a girl of about seventeen who had a lump in her breast, and he was trying to find out the history.

"How long have you had it?" he asked, chalk poised to write the time up on the board.

"I don't know, doctor," she said shyly.

"When did you notice it first hurting?"

"It doesn't hurt, doctor."

"How did you discover it then?" The surgeon was getting irritated.

"I didn't, doctor, it was my boyfriend in the cinema the other night. He told me about it." It was all we could do to strain our laughter.

Sometimes, too, the tables would be turned on the clinician. A woman was supposed to be having a Ryle's tube passed down into her stomach for a specimen of her stomach juices and the student and house surgeon were vainly trying to do it, but she only retched and spat it out when it touched her throat. The sister of the ward tried and was no more successful when the physician in charge of the case came in.

"What haven't you got down yet?" he demanded. "Here, give it to me. I'll show you." And he took the tube and began passing it down her nose which is another way of doing it, and the patient then swallows the tube. Now he was pushing down more and more and was just saying, "There you are, you see it's quite easy?" when he saw we were all laughing. The woman had not swallowed the tube but was pulling it out of her mouth as fast as he was pushing it down her nose! The doctor laughed himself then and walked away saying, "I leave it to you, only get that specimen somehow."

Of the passing of Ryle's tubes I had quite a lot of practice. One time while in Basingstoke I had read a new book by John Fulton on the localization in the brain of different physiological functions of the body, and one of these was a connection between a certain area stimulated by an electric current and the production of excess stomach juices. At once it occurred to me that this was why statistics showed that persons with responsible jobs causing worry were those most likely to have peptic ulcers. If so stopping worry by sleep would cure them.

Back in Dublin I talked to this same young clinician about this and he suggested my experimenting with the idea. So having permission from the respective physicians and with the patients' own consent, I began a series of experiments consisting of putting a Ryle's tube down at night, giving the patient two Soneryl tablets to ensure sound sleep and then drawing off a specimen of juices through the tube with a syringe every two hours. Their day time fractional test meal had already been done and in the case of duodenal ulcers the acid content of the stomach juices was always found to be very high. Now from these experiments I found that during a deep sleep it went down to nil or very low, but if the patient did not sleep well, if he preferred to try without sleeping tablets, it was as high as in daytime.

Finally after doing thirteen of these I got permission from the Professor of Medicine, who was an honorary at my hospital, to try treating a case which had come in, very ill indeed, with both a duodenal and a gastric ulcer and who was then unfit for operation. After three weeks sleeping all day and night except when he was wakened for meals of a high protein diet, his duodenal ulcer had gone, viewed radiographically, and his gastric ulcer remained but very small. He left the hospital delighted and returned to work. Nine months later he returned because of pain and vomiting and this time they operated, the X-ray having shown a return of the gastric ulcer but no sign of the duodenal. A partial gastrectomy was done and a healed scar was noted on the duodenum.

Things move slowly in Ireland, just as they do in the East. Even this evidence did not motivate anyone to take up the matter. But some weeks after, another patient of the Professor who had been treated for some time on the old alkaline and milk diet method and who was no better, demanded that he should be allowed to sleep his ulcer away too, since he had heard of the first case. The Professor grinned at me as we did the round and the man spoke thus.

"If you want to try you can have him," he said, and so I got my second case. It was just as successful, being a duodenal ulcer and not gastric. After three weeks an X-ray showed no sign of the ulcer which had been visible before and his abdomen was no longer tender as it had been.

But it was time for me to go out of residence and I could not pursue the matter any further then. At the Professor's suggestion I wrote up my experiments and two cases for the *Irish Medical Journal* and it was published the term before I qualified. Later I learned that the French and the Russians were also working on the same idea.

Now we had to do a month with each of the specialists, the anesthetist, the E.N.T. man, the ophthalmologist, and dermatologist and the gynecologist. The latter was an ex–Master of the Rotunda and his daughter was in our year and while she was at the hospital with him she always called him "sir," as all the honoraries were called by all students. I enjoyed my month on with him but loathed the tonsillectomies with the E.N.T. man and skins did not interest me at all.

There came a patient up one day who had had a Caesarian done at the Rotunda some months before and who had gone blind while under the anesthetic, having had toxemia of pregnancy. She was warned to have no more children. Then the ophthalmologist who was a cousin of the gynecologist suggested bringing her in to the hospital for examination to see if her eyes were beyond hope. So she came up from the country and then it was found she was pregnant again. They decided to keep her in for full term and she was with us five months.

Annie became a favorite of the ward for she was always cheerful and her big brown eyes, monumental to look at but quite sightless, would turn to the door as one of us who looked after her came in. After the operation and delivery of a boy she returned to her own home, since her blindness was beyond cure.

I passed the Almoner in the corridor one day about a month before Christmas. She asked if I had had any news of Annie since she left but I had not and she told me that she knew she was in a bad way for her husband was out of work as an un-discharged TB and she had six children. Her parents considered she had married beneath her and had repudiated her utterly. I passed on but slowly an idea formed and I went to talk to a girl student who had also been on with the gynecologist and had become quite attached to the patient. I suggested we might have a whip round and collect some Christmas fare for the family. She thought it a good idea and promised to make a big cake and ice it. So then I sought out the honoraries and the other students who had been concerned with her and altogether collected five pounds. Going shopping a few days before Christmas I bought a large hunk of beef, a big plum pudding, tinned fruit and vegetable, dates, nuts, chocolate and sweets, jam, butter and everything suitable for Yuletide. Finally with what was left I visited Woolworths and bought something for each child, all boys, a box of soldiers, a snakes and ladders game, a paint box and book, a story book and a rattle for the newest baby. There was a little left for some turned down stockings and a tie for the husband and handkerchiefs for Annie. These last two were a poor choice due to my lack of knowledge of poverty.

On Christmas Eve I was due to go to Belfast to stay with friends for the day and I went via Cavan county where she lived, in the baby Renault car I had by now bought. It was snowing lightly and bitterly cold by the time I arrived and sought directions as to where Blind Annie lived. I was directed to a white washed cottage in a field and left the car on the road to cross over the powdered snow. I was met by a youngish man with rosy cheeks and two small boys and I asked again for Annie. They took me to the door and there she was turning her blind eyes to see who was coming.

"Hallo, Annie!" I said, and at once her face broke into a smile.

"It's the doctor," she cried and welcomed me in. The fire with its green twigs was blown up into smoke and tea made and she took down from a shelf half a loaf and the remnants of a pot of jam. The husband apologized for the scanty fare saying they had been saving up for Christmas, but it was obvious that this was all they had and there would have been no Christmas if we had not made the effort. Knowing what was in the car I ate freely, as the two boys eyed the disappearing bread wistfully.

"Where are the other two boys?" I asked, "I heard you had four big ones."

"They're in bed in the other room," said the husband, "we've only enough clothes for two to be up at once. These will go to bed this afternoon." And we had not been able to raise any boys' clothes!

I now told them what I had come for and the boys' faces gaped incredulously and doubtless four little ears were straining from the bed in the other room. They came with me to the car and helped to carry over the three big boxes. Two I opened up and showed them the contents, meat, pudding, and all the good things and the third I said was to be kept for tomorrow morning. It was the box of presents and the cake the girl student had made.

I left them all almost in tears, staring dumbly at the boxes and as I drove on up to Belfast I felt that this had been a worthwhile Christmas at last, the way Christmases were meant to be. In my student days I had at least come into contact with real poverty, both while on the district from the Rotunda and in this case; though as yet I had had no experience of it myself.

But what of my social life by this time and what of my relations with my former friends and acquaintances? After re-registration we had decided that only those who were old and firm friends should be allowed to know. I went to Folkestone only once and then to put the house in order when Toto and Daisy wished to return to it at the end of the war. At that time it was still a desolate town and my main job was to cut away the jungle which had once been a garden in order to get to the house and make both back and front entrance usable, and to clean and air the rooms a little. It had suffered no damage, nor had Folkestone itself, oddly enough except for a small area near the harbor and fish-market. That weekend I met only Mr. Whyte whom I sought out and I camped in the sitting room, then left again before my aunts returned. They agreed it would be better not to come to Folkestone again in case I was recognized. Publicity must be avoided at all cost.

Having not had enough income to live on as a student I had decided to raise capital each year and when I had finished my course I would have nothing left but an earning capacity which should, however, keep me out of all difficulties. Auntie Daphne had died in an internment camp in Italy during the war and left me 500 pounds with which I first bought a new motorcycle and later that baby Renault car, trading in the bike in part exchange. Also it seemed good business to invest capital on buying a house and letting part of it while living in one story as a flat. And this I did so that I was assured of a weekly income.

Now I could have the sort of sitting room-study I had long dreamed of. Books everywhere on shelves I made myself and leather chairs and sofa, a dining room table and a bureau, with my rowing photographs on the wall and my cups, as they accumulated, on the mantle piece which was brick over a brick fireplace. The second room was a bedroom with two beds so that I could put up a friend should any want to stay. In one corner of the sitting room was a small table with gin, sherry and Irish whiskey for visitors. When I first was introduced to alcohol in Oxford I had vowed to myself that although I would drink I would never allow myself to become drunk and incapable, having the example of my father before me.

Shunning temptation in a teetotaler's pledge was not the way. To indulge without becoming a slave was. And this vow I now renewed and kept even when I went to sea where drink was cheap and plentiful.

At the end of my first term I had gone to Belfast with the crew for a regatta and a fellow medical student who was coxing asked me to stay with him which I did along with three others of the crew. Both his parents were doctors, a most delightful family, united and offering of itself to those who were homeless. This was a special feature of Christmas there, for the dinner table was surrounded by those who would have dined alone had they not been invited. And thither I went each Christmas thereafter. Indeed I had a standing invitation after my first visit to go when I would.

It was this boy's mother, who was much more nearly my contemporary than he was, whose father had been Bobby's trustee and whose mother had disapproved of his being with "that woman," Mrs. Hearne. On my first visit I was asked if I was related to Bobby and dutifully denied it, but two years later when I knew them all well enough to trust them implicitly I admitted the relationship and it was then that I learned of this and of other things connected with his childhood in Ireland.

But I made no other close friends among my fellow students until my last year when an ex–service man from Wales joined my hospital and I offered to let him share my flat, an arrangement which worked very well as it transpired, since he was the company, which I lacked so much, of someone who had seen something of the world and not a young enthusiast just out of school.

At first I had to force myself to take part in certain social functions, for I was shy and the mental scars of past events were still felt. Indeed, for the first two years I felt a real fear that I would wake up one morning and find myself back in the garage, of which I sometimes dreamed; that this was all too good to be true. I went to an occasional dance held by the College Societies around Christmas, notably the Biological Association which had a big affair at the end of the Michaelmas term and which was a medical student society, and the dance was frequented by students and doctors. I early found I had to acquire a white tie and tails and liked the look of myself in them—I, who had long since refused to wear the evening dress which had been considered appropriate for me before. Not that I could dance, having forgotten what I had learned at the dancing classes as a child, except for the waltz which I remembered. In those days the foxtrot and the tango were only just coming in and the polka, the waltz, the gallop and Sir Roger had chiefly composed our lessons, dances hardly seen by this time. Before I would never go to a dance for I would not have a man put his arm around me but now I made what I could of them and enjoyed the occasional evening. But partners were kind and helped me out, not all the girl students being able to dance well themselves anyway. With girls one had to be careful. No one seemed to suspect anything and I developed something of a reputation of being a woman-hater, since I made a point of treating them in a rather rough brotherly fashion, and sheered off if any showed any signs of being interested. One must not lead a girl on if one could not give her children. That was the basis of my ethics. An evening's flirting at a dance was one thing and a relief—but no more.*

The Biological Association also held weekly meetings at which a member read a paper and there were annual prizes for the best in various groups. Each year I read a paper, wearing my Oxford M.A. gown which had belonged to Jimmy[†] to deliver it. For the first three years I won the Junior prize annually, for students under four years standing. Then followed the bronze medal, and for the last two years the silver medal, the last paper being my account of my sleep therapy experiments. And the last but one, on the hypothalamus, was also published in the *Irish Medical Journal*.

When not doing examinations in which one had to reproduce the textbook, I was on my own ground, and in addition entered for an All-Ireland student's essay competition, flaying the Welfare State in general and nationalized medicine in particular, and winning the prize for my own University as well as the extra prize given for the best of the five University winners. But I never did well in examinations, only just scraping through each time.

My last visit to Rooksdown was in 1949, and then I began those cycling holidays on the continent which continued until 1956 whenever leave from my ship made a trip possible. In 1949 I went with a Nigerian medical student of my year, coal black, with a poetic and mystic streak in him. We took [a] train to Dijon and cycled down the Rhone to Marseilles, seeing to my delight the famous Roman remains of Orange and Vienna, for I had seen none such before, although my classical training had left me with a keen interest in its archaeology. Then we rode along the coast to Narbonne and took the train through the Pyrenees and finally cycled up the Loire to Paris. It was my first foreign excursion and the widening of the vistas appealed to me, circumscribed as I had been heretofore.

* Added here by hand: "Yet often I felt resentful that I should always be alone, and never have [several words crossed out and illegible]."

† Jimmy McKie, Dillon's philosophy tutor from Brasenose College, Oxford.

We were out three weeks and during that time, camping and eating once a day in restaurants, I did not shave. On my return I thought my beard showed a promising shape and left it to see what would happen. Eventually I wore it in a King George V style, and it proved invaluable, since I found that with it I could safely visit Folkestone and no one could guess who I was—or had been.

This trip set the pattern for future ones which became more astringent and took the form of an ascetic exercise. I was myself puzzled to know what made me go on them, because they were only enjoyable in retrospect. Days of fighting head winds, nights in the open battling with mosquitoes, only one meal a week now in a restaurant and the rest cooked over a campfire— this was to be the form my holidays took. On the carrier would be slung a blanket, a plastic cape, two billy cans and a towel and a sweater, and in my belt was a sheath knife. One did not need much more and all weight took its toll.

When I was at sea and earning well I took my old garage friend G., with whom I had renewed acquaintance after his discharge from the Navy, and showed him the sights of Italy. On the first night after we had had a hard day's pedaling and could find no good camping terrain, we parked under a bridge where there were more rocks than grass. G. sank down and said plaintively: "You know, Mike, this is supposed to be a *holiday!*" But soon he also became infected with the idea and followed so eagerly that he came again the next time.

Having changed my names I had decided to drop the Laurence, too much like the old name, and use Michael, which was often reduced to Mike, and in due course I discovered I was about the fourth Michael Dillon there was in Ireland, at least of those who were known, and there were probably many others "born to blush unseen" among the peat bogs and the white washed cottages.

My cousin Joan visited me in my flat once. Before the war she had been a shy school girl and I had not seen her since. Now as an ex–Lance corporal of the A.T.S. there seemed to be nothing she did not know about the world and its ways. She stayed two nights, I sleeping on the floor of the sitting room while she had the bedroom, and then came a furious letter from her mother, Auntie Evie, to say she should not have stayed there with me now; it was most improper. We neither of us cared!

But Evie was slowly dying, though we did not know it then. Maudie and she, identical twins that they were, had each developed cancer within three weeks of each other, at least the diagnosis was made within that period.

Maudie had it in the axilla and Evie in the breast, which had been removed but the cells had already spread and were beginning to block the lymphatics of her arm so that it was assuming elephantine proportions. Maudie died the year before I took my finals and left me one third of her property, which amounted some £20,000, sharing it with Bobby and Joan, for her brother Leslie had been killed in the war. He had joined the R.A.F. and gone to Cranwell from school and when called up saw active service from the start. Before the blitzes he was on a reconnaissance flight over the coast of France when he was shot down just before his twenty-first birthday. His body was recovered and buried over there.

This bequest changed the uncertain future for now there would still be something when I had qualified, and I exchanged the motorcycle for the baby Renault. In the Easter vacation before my finals I toured Ireland in it with a very dear friend from Bristol, a clergyman, some thirty years older than myself, whom I had met at the beginning of the war and so who had known me before in the time of my troubles. Although he had not been able to offer much material help in those days, one could always tell him anything and he would never be shocked. His understanding and his compassion were immense, and his learning was no less. When, later, I broke it to him that I had become a Buddhist monk he wrote back and said he was sure I knew what I was doing and wished me happiness, orthodox clergyman though he was.*

On this holiday, we set out down to Wexford, along to Cork, through Killarney and Tralee, up to Galway, across Connemara after a visit to Athlone and Clonmacnoise, then over the border to Enniskerry and on to Belfast where I took him to lunch with my doctor friends, and home again. All in three and a half days. But then you can run across Ireland in three hours in a good car. Clonmacnoise was his contribution to the trip. I had

* The clergyperson referenced here is the Reverend Canon A. R. Millbourn of Bristol Cathedral. The canon remained in contact with Dillon / Jivaka for the rest of D/J's life, receiving letters from him up until shortly before his death in 1962. Canon Millbourn also wrote a preface to Roberta Cowell's 1954 memoir *Roberta Cowell's Story*, writing, "if her book brings me into touch with others who have had comparable experiences, the obligation will be greater still. There must be many such; and if nothing else has been gained, the openness of such a story as is told in these pages could be of immense help to them in their own struggle, which in the nature of things is likely to be a single-handed one. Reticence is a very desirable thing, but secretiveness can sometimes be a very dangerous one" (ix).

not heard of it. But it seemed it was the last home of classical learning in Europe before the Danes destroyed that too, after all the other monasteries had fallen. When later I was in India I discovered that the Moslem hate let loose against the Buddhist monasteries and universities coincided in time precisely with that of the Danish destruction of the Christians. As Clonmacnoise fell so fell Nalanda, one of the largest Buddhist universities, and the last to be leveled, both in the same century. Is it coincidence or is there something outside that causes men to act thus, that sends waves of different types of destruction over the face of the earth? An analysis of history would suggest that such coincidences are rather frequent to be passed off as chance.

Now before us was the last great hurdle, the Finale examination in Medicine and Surgery at the end of the summer term. Yearly we had exams to pass usually three at a time, and in the previous term we had had the smaller ones of Ophthalmology, Psychological medicine, Forensic medicine and the bigger one of Gynecology and Obstetrics. I only passed that one by luck. In the viva just before me had gone in the daughter of the gynecologist previously mentioned. As she came out in the moment's pause while they were marking her effort, I asked what she was asked.

"Insufflation of tubes," she said. I was horrified—I knew next to nothing about it. Then she whispered an invaluable tip: the point at which to stop inflating if you do not want to do damage. Next moment I was called in. And sure enough that question was asked and it was the only one on insufflation I knew the answer to, but the all-important one. But for the tip I would surely have failed!

For Finals we had written, practical and a viva. The practical would be on real patients at any one of the hospitals. No one knew till the morning to which hospital he would be sent. This was to prevent students checking cases before the examination. In Surgery I had luck again. Indeed, these sorts of exams depend largely on luck. There was a shortage of patients and I had a straight appendix for my primary and the external examiner was an Oxford man. There were always two examiners, one invited from another university. I was in the habit of wearing my old university tie with the coat of arms, the book and triple crown of Oxford, for examinations for luck, and he happened to be wearing the same. The result was, when he came round, he started asking me about Oxford instead of my case until the Trinity examiner arrived and then he hurriedly asked me about appendectomies. The key question was about postoperative treatment and I knew the answer they wanted. The minor case was hand infections, so one way and another I was fortunate and scraped past the fifty percent together with the papers' marks.

In the Medical it was my curious innate honesty that got me through on the minor case and a well-developed sympathy with patients on the major. Once again through shortage I was given as a major a patient who was really too ill to be pulled around in an examination and I was warned to go easy with him. As so much a patient myself I always managed to get on well with the sick and he told me in a whisper his history. The history is all-important and many students fail because they rub the patient up the wrong way and he or she refuses to tell them anything. But this man was an advanced heart case and all went well. The examiners did not want to pull him about either.

The minor, however, reduced me to despair. A woman had vomited and fallen down unconscious while cooking the breakfast and when recovered was paralyzed in both legs. On first hearing this one would say a subarachnoid hemorrhage. But on examination she produced the impossible situation of having her plantar and ankle reflexes present and her knee reflexes gone. The examiner came round.

"Your name? Dillon? Yes, well, what's your diagnosis, Dillon?"

"There isn't one, sir," I said miserably, "she is contrary to all the textbooks."

The examiner smiled. "You'll often find that in the course of your practice," he said. "Well, tell me what you've found."

I gave him the history and ended with, "The plantar and ankle reflexes are present and the knee one is gone. It's impossible."

He looked at me disbelievingly, for it was impossible. You could have it the other way round but not the upper reflexes present and lower absent.

"And the abdominal?" he asked.

"They're absent too, sir, but then she's over fifty." (They normally disappear with time.)

"Let's see." And he sat on the bed and began to test her while I waited in agony lest he found results different from mine.

"Yes, you're quite right," he said. "What do you suppose it is?"

"Some sort of cerebral hemorrhage, but I can't say where." I said. The second examiner now joined us and confirmed the findings. They nodded and left me in the belief that I must have failed.

I passed! It seemed that the hospital doctors themselves did not know exactly what the cause was but had postulated possible multiple minor spinal hemorrhages on top of an initial cerebral one. The student who came after me said immediately "Subarachnoid hemorrhage" and failed.

The results were out. We celebrated in the traditional way with whiskey, beer, gin and anything going, but as always I stopped as soon as I began to see things were not quite so clear cut as they normally looked. Next morning I had to tell myself that I was at last a doctor, and for many mornings after, since it seemed so unlikely. My life had been so strange and at one time so impossible that now as a respectable member of the community and accepted at my face value, it was too good, far too good to be true. Within me I felt an intense gratitude and devotion to that, whatever it was, an Absolute, a Father-God or what you will, who had brought me out of the slough of despond on to level ground from which the far-off hills could be seen to be green. I went into a church and gave thanks.

CHAPTER 7

Resident Medical Officer

I naturally expected, as also did all my friends, that I would be one of those four who would be given a house appointment in the Royal City of Dublin hospital where we had worked. It could only take four out of the many applicants, but previously no other student had done any research work during his course or had papers published before he was qualified. Great was the shock therefore, and blow to my pride when it was announced that the four highest marks in the examination had been accepted, and of these I was certainly not one. Even one or two of the doctors thought it was unfair. Now I did not know what to do. I cycled away from the hospital, my elation turned to gloom. Where should I go? All the teaching hospitals would be full of their own men and Belfast students would go to various provincial hospitals in the North.

There was one small hospital in the north of Dublin having but fifty beds and requiring a single R.M.O.* who was house physician and surgeon

* RMO stands for resident medical officer. Such positions could have greater flexibility and cover more than one location but could be compensated less well, as Dillon/Jivaka indicates.

in one as well as attendant on specialist clinics each week. Here one would learn much more, having varied experience, but the pay was then only £1 a week. The man in charge of it was the surgeon from my own hospital who had let me do my first appendectomy. I went to see him, therefore, and asked for the job and was readily accepted, since there was not much demand for such small rate of pay. (It was raised to £2 a week after I had been there a short time [after learning] that it was quite out of line with other jobs in the British Isles.)

But first one must have a holiday and the then-Resident was willing to stay on another month while I went on one of my cycle trips, this time to Italy. I had a great desire to see Rome and Pompeii. As yet G. was not available for such a holiday, being married with a young son and struggling to make a living in London, so I went alone, taking the train to Naples and from there riding out first to Pompeii.

This place fascinated me. Despite noisy American tourists, the deathly quiet was undisturbed. And one wandered up the streets of that city of the dead, trying to imagine it as it had been before the fateful eruption of Vesuvius on August 24, 79 A.D., about which Pliny the Younger wrote such a vivid description and which I had read during my days at Oxford, never dreaming then that I should see the scene for myself.

I went next by the inland road to Rome where the Coliseum and other remains thrilled me, but the modern Roman seemed surprisingly unaware of his ancestry and several people did not know how to direct me to the ruins. Then I followed the coast. Livorno, San Martin, Genoa, Monaco and finally Nice and Cannes, fell before my wheel. The famous Rivieras were seen as cheaply as they could be. One night I pitched camp in a glade belonging to a big hotel at San Martin, and after my supper out of the billy can I strolled over and looked down at the hotel, and counted seventy-two palatial cars parked outside, and wondered how much they were being stung for their night's lodging and whether it was really any more comfortable than mine, with my blanket spread on a grassy bed which I had cut with my sheath knife.

Then back to Dublin to take up hospital life again. The first day one felt as new and strange as a boy at his first boarding school. Before one "belongs" one feels out of it, the only person who does not know exactly what to do and when to do it. I was to have the same feeling again on my first day at Rizong Monastery when I went to Ladakh.

But soon the routine was established. There were two visiting surgeons and so two operating days a week for outpatients admitted, as well as emergencies for which one or another surgeon would have to come over. And each of the other days there was a clinic, whether for skins, eyes, or women's diseases, although we did not normally do midwifery, but the gynecologist sometimes operated on his cases there. Yet I was fortunate in having a baby delivered while in residence. A woman booked for the Rotunda had gone into labor while on the bus and the conductor had become nervous and put her off at our hospital door. I admitted her, informing the gynecologist by phone and, receiving permission, delivered the baby in the theater in due course. The matron said afterwards that I carried that baby round the women's ward as proudly as if I had been its father!

In Ireland there is, or was not at that time, any system of occupational therapy in the hospitals except for the tuberculosis ones. We had an outdoor hut of five beds for tubercular patients in on long term, but otherwise we were not registered as a T.B. hospital and we did not take open chest cases. The sight of the patients lying in their beds with nothing to do but think and talk of their ailments gave me an idea. At Rooksdown occupational therapy was a major contribution to the cures and I had learned a variety of handicrafts while there. Now it seemed a good idea to start the system here. If I could raise some capital from the honoraries to buy materials, it might be possible to sell the products and so buy more materials and keep everyone busy and their minds off their bodies.

The surgeon in charge thought it was a good idea and gave me something as also did the other honoraries and I set out to buy leather and tools, embroidery silks and cloths to embroider, knitting wool, and parchment for lampshades. The women, of course, could embroider and knit and make children's frocks without help. And the leatherwork was taken up easily by the men who learned to punch holes and thread and stitch, to make wallets, purses, handbags and belts. A very popular line was the cowboy belt which I designed myself, with pockets that were thief proof, and with a sheath for a knife and loops for cartridges (or other commodities!) and swivels on either side and with a large buckle. Then on visiting days we would put the goods out on a table in the hall and offer them for sale. The response surpassed all belief. Not only was I able to continue to buy more and better materials but in the one year I was there we turned over a clear profit of £100.

It began slowly but by Christmas there was enough in the kitty to take all up-patients to the Pantomime, by arrangement with the manager of the theater, for a couple of wheelchairs had to stay in the aisle. Taxis took the others there and back and for those who were confined to bed there was a big tea.

Next it seemed a good idea to fit all the beds with head phones so that patients could listen to the wireless when they liked, and they were linked with the radio set in the nurses' common-room. The four wards had to be wired and this took up a good portion of our money. But there was still some over.

Now among the long-term patients in the TB hut was a young fellow of eighteen who had been there three years with a TB hip and abscess. He was a very quiet, respectful youth, quite unlike the other four who were of the peasantry, but also very shy and would hardly talk. In the spring X-rays showed that the disease was quiescent if not conquered and it was decided to discharge him. Now normally the parents would be informed and they would bring his clothes and he would go home with them. But this lad had no parents, he had no known relatives and indeed did not even own the name he had been given. For he had been a foundling near some village to the south and had been brought up by foster parents to whom he had been farmed out by the County Council which was paying for him to be maintained in hospital.

When he had first been admitted after a year in another place he was only fifteen. During his time in bed he had grown to more than six foot and he had no clothes but what the hospital lent him to wear in bed. The council was informed and requested to send the wherewithal to dress him and to equip him completely. They sent £12!

I went to see the manager of a cut-price clothes shop in Dublin and told him the story and asked what he thought he could do to help us in this case. He agreed to make a suit for seven pounds and with the rest I bought two shirts, two of each underwear, socks and a cheap mackintosh. There was nothing for shoes which the Matron and myself subscribed between us.

When he was up and dressed the next thing was to socialize him. During all his formative years he had been an invalid, waited on and without friends except for fellow patients, and he had exactly two possessions of his own: a cheap ball-point pen some visitor had given him and an old, broken pair of shoes which he had brought with him and were naturally far too small. He had been one of the best embroiderers, too, being neat and quick with his fingers.

But he was most painfully shy and nothing would make him speak. He wanted to hide away in a corner or sit on his bed with those he knew. I started taking him down the town in my car but when I made him get out to go and look at the shops he shrunk against the wall and would not move. Then I thought of taking another patient too who was getting up and who had at one time worked in England and was not in the least shy. Having a companion gave him more confidence.

One Saturday afternoon I decided to go to the pictures and to take these two with me. Johnnie sat in his seat his eyes glued to the screen throughout, thrilled with the film which was Lytton's *Last Days of Pompeii*. I told him I had been there and seen the ruins and he murmured his usual "Yes, sir," which was the modicum of his conversations with me as a rule.

That evening I went back to my flat and took out a book called *The Destruction and Resurrection of Pompeii and Herculaneum*. It was an archaeological and historical work, nothing light about it, except the translation of Pliny's vivid account of the eruption and this I gave him to read, marking the three relevant pages. Two days later he gave me the book back and to my astonishment he said he had read it all.

Here was a boy who had nothing to read for four years but the odd western or romance that the weekly visit of the hospital librarian brought him and who had had the minimum of education, reading a book of that caliber.

"Tomorrow afternoon," I said, "I will take you to my flat in Ballsbridge and let you choose some books to read. I have about nine hundred."

He smiled with pleasure as he gave his quiet "Thank you, sir."

And when I showed him my books he picked out three, two on ancient Greece and one on Egyptology. I was amazed. Then he spoke:

"I am interested in this sort," he said.

Thereafter when he had finished his books he would take them back and change them and soon he had read all of such that I had and had gone on to the popular scientific variety. This made me think.

If during those long years in hospital he had been reading he could have educated himself considerably. With what was left of the money from the sales of the patients' products I decided to make a bookcase with glass doors and found an educational library, so that any who came in the future could learn what they wanted. Then, whenever there was any more money to spare I went to the second hand bookshops to see what I could buy. *Teach Yourself* loomed largely, naturally, but also popular works on science, astronomy, music, and as many of the great classics as I could find, together with books on literature and grammar, with French, German and Latin, and shorthand, book-keeping and other trades to balance. Whenever a patient said he or she was interested in a certain subject I tried to find a book on that. They had only to tell the sister of the ward and she would look in the bookcase to find one to satisfy them.

Meanwhile the honoraries had been very pleased with the way the morale of the patients had gone up and it seemed as if their time in bed was reduced a little as their minds were better occupied than they had been before. Indeed the surgeon said that when he came into a ward it was more like a factory. The table would be covered in leather and cloth which the up-patients would cut out for those in bed, notably Johnnie who was very energetic about helping those who were sick, now that he was about again. With them he felt no shyness and he could be seen piloting a blind old man to the lavatory or helping George to practice walking with his artificial legs.

With summer now approaching I began taking long-term patients out for runs in my Renault and wondered why members of the hospital committee never thought to do that when they all ran cars. Those who lie in bed day after day and see only the same limited landscape feel a happiness out of all proportion to the little trouble involved, when they are suddenly taken from the prison of their room and allowed to see once again trees, flowers, people and shops—or the sea, which was but ten miles away and several picnics we had on the cliff at Malahide, taking our tea with us. It was thus that Johnnie saw the sea for the first time in his life.

It seemed he was quite out of touch with the most ordinary things. He had never used a telephone or sent a telegram or seen a play. I took him to the Gate theater for his introduction to the theatrical world. By now he was coming out of his shell a little and would reply if spoken to but never volunteered anything on his own.

For a further experiment in civilizing him I took him to Belfast one weekend to my doctor friends there, watching carefully what others did, and although at first during dinner, knife and fork disappeared under the table between each mouthful, he soon saw the way we used them and copied. They liked him and he saw a proper home for the first time where people lived in comfort and a family in its normal setting. There was something of breeding about the boy who was certainly by no means a peasant and I concluded he must have been the product of a landed squire and a farmer's girl or maid servant who had abandoned the baby lest her disgrace be discovered—if she had not done away with herself as well thereafter. He had certainly good blood in his veins.

The problem now was what was to be done with him. His former foster parents had had other children of their own since he had left and there was no room for this young giant in their tiny white-washed cottage. Nor was there any rehabilitation scheme in Ireland and no firm would employ him with his medical history. Moreover he still walked with a limp and was not fit for manual labor which alone was open to him.

It seemed that he must go to England where there were opportunities, so I wrote to my good friend G., now a little better situated, and asked if he could get him a job in the town where he worked. So successful was this overture that in no time it was arranged that Johnnie should fly over and stay with G. himself who was at that time a grass-widower for six months while his wife and their child were on a visit to her parents who were not English and lived abroad.

He also found him a job with a wine firm, bottling and labeling at £5 a week, a fortune to the orphan and he paid for his keep. He and G., both of similar origins, got on well together. He had started a new life and he would make something of it. When G.'s wife returned and he had to go into digs, he came down on the next Christmas day with his arms full of expensive presents for all of them. And when G. remonstrated with him for spending his money on them when he needed it for himself, his reply in that soft Irish accent of his was:

"Not at all! Sure it's wonderful to know the pleasure there is in giving!"

Not all people have discovered that pleasure yet although it is there for everyone to sample. Up to then he had nothing to give. It had been a shock to me that day I had discovered that a lad of eighteen could exist who only had two possessions in the world, and I had gone back to my flat and looked around at all the useless things there were: pictures, silver cups, ornaments, a wardrobe full of clothes and so on. How could one own all these things when there was a boy with absolutely nothing? Not that he had the right to demand anything, but I had a duty to give. This is the difference between Communism and Christianity.

It was as the result of all this that was born the idea that I pursued for the next six years while at sea of giving one tenth, or a tithe of my pay-off after each voyage, to that clergyman friend in Bristol to use for any struggling students who needed ready aid. He was on the committee for special grants to such but this met only periodically and had many strings attached to its charity. This was to be for immediate distribution in any case which came to his notice of real urgent need. A girl who had won a scholarship but whose parents could not afford to pay for books, club subscriptions and the other necessities of college life, was the first to be helped by the "kitty" we formed, and she took a first class and was sent to a French University for a year post-graduate, and so were we repaid.

Another lad who had been born in the slums of St. Pancras and who had seen every form of vice by the age of twelve, had used his time well during his spell in the Navy during and after the war, educating himself by means of the Seafarers Education Society, and he had even taught himself Latin. After his discharge he changed his name to that of the Commander of his ship who bore a famous one, and started at a theological college intent on taking Holy Orders. After one year his money was finished and he could not pay his terminal fees. They gave him grace for one term and then reluctantly told him he would have to leave if no money was forthcoming. He had heard of the clergyman who administered the grants trust but he would have to have waited for the committee to meet and it would have been too late even if they agreed to help him.

"Can you do with twenty pounds down?" asked the clergyman and the boy nearly broke down. Next Sunday he returned and insisted on working in the Canon's garden all day to show his gratitude. Thus was the kitty distributed and after each voyage replenished again. My own feeling of gratitude for being able to live a normal life and to be in the Merchant Navy at all was in part assuaged by this, for I felt I could never be grateful enough to those who had come into my life and helped me when there seemed no solution to my own problem or for that Force which seemed to be pushing me along to an unknown goal. But it was the case of Johnnie which first gave the impetus. Those who thirst for knowledge and can find none through poverty or circumstances, these were the ones I wanted to help most.

This year as R.M.O. was eventful for another quite distinct event. At Christmas I received a present from someone of a book. It was entitled *In Search of the Miraculous* by P. D. Ouspensky, of whom I had never heard until that time.* Lying on my bed in the little cottage in the garden where the house surgeon lived, I read it with interest although much of it was beyond my comprehension. Yet when it was finished it seemed that at last here was a man who had put one foot outside the circle in which all other philosophers were milling, for I had long since lost patience with philosophical works and now could not bring myself to read them. They went round and round the same problems but this man had broken away. He had penetrated into that dark room on the threshold of which I had felt I

---

* P. D. Ouspensky (1878–1947), a Russian mathematician, is known for teaching and extending the spiritual system of the Russian mystic, composer, and philosopher George I. Gurdjieff (1866–1949).

was standing when I wrote the chapter on Free-Will in my own little book which had sold out its edition without making much of a mark.

I read it through a second time and then put it away to allow it to simmer inside me. His point about negative emotion which must be shed struck me as all too true, as also the way we revel in our self-pity. This of course he had learned from Gurdjieff, his Guru, but of Gurdjieff I had not heard either. Meanwhile I procured his other two books but did not find them so striking as that one.* They had been written before he met Gurdjieff.

My year as R.M.O. was drawing to a close and I must begin to think of what to do next. In a way I was sorry; I had enjoyed it once over my disappointment at not getting into my teaching hospital and probably I had more experience here than I would have [had] there. The hospital being small was matey, as it were, run with the minimum of rules and that senior nursing staff were all friends who had trained together and among them were two pairs of sisters.

I had not been there a month before the matron had died on me. She had had a cerebral hemorrhage and lingered for three or four days and never recovered consciousness again. Then it was I had my first experience of an Irish Roman Catholic funeral with its wake. She was laid out in her "sister of Mary" robe, whatever that was, in pale blue, on her bed in the room next to my dining room. And for the twenty-four hours before her funeral she was not left alone for a minute. Her relatives even had their meals in with the body, which was to be taken to the church to lie in state overnight and the service would then be the following morning.

Following Protestant custom I arrived for the funeral cortege in a dark grey suit and black tie to find that everyone else was attired in their usual colors! As we followed the coffin up the road the crowd was talking and joking, very different from the solemn funerals I had attended before for various members of my own family. The next morning I went with the head sister to the church and found the funeral service was to be held in a side aisle and a wedding ceremony in the center aisle, since someone had made a muddle of the timings and neither side would give way. The service was gabbled at great speed in Latin and then we all repaired back to the hospital where we were regaled with sherry and cakes. It was all most unusual to my insular mind!

---

* Dillon/Jivaka notes these books as *Tertium Organum* (1920) and *New Model of the Universe* (1931).

A new matron had to be selected and I was in the position of hearing both sides of the matter—from the head surgeon who was thinking of choosing someone from outside and from the nursing staff who would all have resigned if a stranger was brought in who might start to alter the traditional ways we had of doing things and bringing it into line with other hospitals as regards rules. It would have been Rooksdown all over again. So I took an opportunity of offering *gratis* my advice which was to promote the theater sister to Matron, who had the allegiance of the whole staff and had been at the hospital for many years and would therefore keep things as they had been. He listened and so it happened.

Operations I saw many of and was allowed to do some when the surgeon was there, and minor surgery I could, of course, do on my own. And medical cases were many and various. One old woman was put into hospital for a fortnight by her family since she was bedridden and they wished to go on holiday. I was told she was a heart case but could not find much wrong and one day I suggested she might like to sit up in a chair. So I lifted her into the chair and let her look out of the window. Her heart showed no ill effects. Then we started taking a turn round the ward before going back to bed, and still she seemed quite well and she got up every evening. Finally I offered to take her for a run in my car one day. The poor old soul was delighted and was now walking quite freely round the ward with a stick.

Out we went into the country and back again and her heart ticked on quite normally. Then the day came for her sons and daughter-in-law to fetch her and when they came she was walking up and down the ward. Their mouths fell open wide.

"But the doctor said she would die if she ever got out of bed even," they told me—a little late as it happened! But she was far from dying and need not have been bedridden for so long. They did not seem pleased at all, oddly enough, and the Matron had to write three times before she got the fees out of them for her two weeks' holiday!

Another old woman of eighty-one fell in love with me and wrote me letters of girlish passion; she must have reached adolescence on the way to her second childhood!

I took two of the nurses to the Biological Association dance that year and we joined up with others and had a good party, but there was not much time for social affairs since one was always on call and if I wanted to go to the cinema or elsewhere it was necessary to leave word where I could be found. The Dublin cinemas were kind to doctors and allowed them to reserve a seat by phone so that they did not have to stand in a queue for a popular film.

Thus, with spring and Johnnie safely away I began to think of the future and decided to see the world at someone else's expense for a year before settling down to the research job I had in mind, something to do with brains, wherever I could find a laboratory that would take me.

I wrote to several shipping companies and was accepted by the P & O– B.I. combine* after an interview and medical examination at which I told no more than was necessary to explain matters, and I was passed as fit.

Assigned to a B.I. ship on the East African run, I was told to do a relief job on a P & O cargo vessel just back from Hong Kong and due to load and unload on the continent first, during which trip it was customary to give the regular surgeon leave. A uniform I would need, and [I] repair[ed] to the naval tailor indicated, who was well versed in fitting out personnel for these illustrious firms whose standards were higher than those of many shipping companies. I was measured for my "blues" and for a mess kit with five pounds' worth of gold braid on red round the sleeves, and [was] sold an enormous quantity of tropical wear, shirts and shorts, number tens, that is tunics buttoning up to the throat with brass buttons and long white trousers, and tropical mess kit. Then there was the cap with the B.I. badge on the front and a blue raincoat. Never had I dreamed I would one day adorn myself in such glad rags!

I went down to Folkestone to stay with the aunts for three days and told them of the new venture. By now they were beyond being surprised at anything and the only protest came from Toto who said I should have joined the Royal Navy since there were no gentlemen in the Merchant, which fact I later found to be quite untrue. My last act was to go out and buy a Merchant Navy tie, with its narrow red, white, and green stripes on blue.

---

* P & O—B.I. Combine refer to the Peninsular and Oriental Steam Navigation Company and the British India Steam Navigation Company. See the first footnote in Chapter 8.

Surgeon M.N.

I was to be not one but six years at sea. One might have known it! From childhood the sea had held a lure for me, and any summer's day not in it I had counted wasted. Now being on it was to have the same attraction. But those six years would make a book in themselves, and to compress them into three short chapters necessitates many omissions.

The first coasting trip on the P&O vessel was to break me in before I joined the B.I. ship with a couple of hundred passengers on board.* This was useful, for as yet I knew no more of ship routine or etiquette than

---

* P&O and BI stand for "Peninsular and Oriental Steam Navigation Company" and "British India Steam Navigation Company," two steam powered shipping companies of the British Merchant Navy. Founded during the mid-nineteenth century, both companies were responsible for empire building through mail contracts and speculative trading between Britain and countries in South and East Asia. When Dillon joined the merchant navy in 1952, P&O and BI were turning from moving mail to passengers and cargo, as tourism was rapidly becoming a booming market.

might be culled from reading *Hornblower* avidly, and that series gave information somewhat out of date!*

It was with timid feelings that I climbed the ship's gangway as she lay in King George V Docks and saw at the top an Indian in what seemed to be Naval ratings uniform. This I later learned was the secunny or Quartermaster. I had been told that the crews of both companies were Indian and that I should learn Hindustani since they were never allowed to speak to the officers in English. So I had come armed with two Hindustani books, neither of which was the slightest bit of use. Either could tell you how to ask "How far is the railway station?" or "How much does this cost?" but neither could tell me how to say: "Are your bowels open?" or "Have you vomited today?" which is much more useful in a surgery!

A passing English youth clad only in shorts picked up my bag and showed me to my cabin, calling a Goanese who said he was my personal servant. The Goanese then proceeded to unpack for me. Never before had I had a personal servant and had always looked after myself, so I sat down in a comfortable armchair and watched his efficiency. My uniform was laid out for me on the bed—no bunk now—and I must put it on for dinner, which would be in a half an hour. Then he left me.

It was a palatial cabin, the most palatial I would ever have as it turned out; the furniture was covered with cheerful chintzes and a broad mahogany desk with many drawers looked a useful asset. There was a long mirror over the dressing table, and in this I gazed with disbelief after adorning myself in my new plumes. Could this really be me? What a long way I had come from those garage days, and longer still from the days of my prized pilot coat and sailor hat. I put on the cap with its white cover and looked again. The three gold stripes on red on the sleeves were embarrassingly glaring, and I felt self conscious at the thought of having to go outside the cabin in this rig. But there, the dinner bell was going and I must find my way to the saloon.

Here I met my brother officers and the Captain, a perfect gentleman who belied my aunt's gloomy announcement that there were none such in the Merchant Navy. They were immediately friendly and anxious to put me at my ease. The Chief Engineer and the C.O. also had their wives with them, and the latter his small daughter.† Two families from the company's

---

* Dillon/Jivaka is referencing C. S. Forrester's novels (1937–1967) about a fictional Royal Navy officer during the Napoleonic Wars.
† CO, or Chief Officer.

office were traveling for their summer holiday, one with a little boy and the other a seventeen-year-old schoolgirl. We would be away about three weeks and were to visit Antwerp, Hamburg, and Rotterdam, to unload and reload cargo for the Far East from whence the ship had just come. It was the Captain's first voyage as master while his Mate (or chief officer as they prefer to call them in the P&O and B.I.) knew the ship well. They had sailed together before in various capacities during their careers at sea.

I went to my bunk that night feeling intensely happy. This was the life for me! I would see the world and become a real sailor. And I now began to wish I had been in a position to go to sea as an apprentice from boyhood, but such wishing was futile. At all events I was intensely grateful for whatever had led me hither and to all those who had made this possible.

Rotterdam, resurrecting from its terrible war devastation, was deeply impressive, and its people were friendly as the Dutch always are at home, whereas in their colonies they were hostile in the extreme. But it was in Antwerp that I first discovered the virtues of the Mission to Seamen, or Flying Angel, for the padre there was a livewire, and did all he could for the seamen who came to his port. Here it was that the Captain developed an attack of shingles across his chest. This can be an incapacitating disease, and he did not want to miss his first long voyage as master. One particular substance injected would bring instant relief, but I could not find it in my dispensary and it was a public holiday in Antwerp. The padre ran me all round the town in his car until we found a hospital who could supply it. Then down to the ship, and the captain had his first injection before nightfall. The next day he was quite happy again, out of pain, although the rash would persist for some time.

And here one morning I felt a great urge to climb the mast to the lookout, doubtless due to my imaginings of myself as a sailor! I went to ask the Old Man his permission. He grinned.

"It's your own bloody silly neck if you want to break it," he said kindly, "Go ahead!" So ahead I went, up and up and up the long thin ladder and then through the lubber's hole, for my courage was insufficient to take me round the outside. At last I stood on the lookout and saw the town lying far and wide about us, and there on the deck like tiny specks the Chief's wife and another lady passenger looking up in fear that I should fall. Beginning to come down from a height is perhaps the worst part, especially if you think about it for too long first. So I did not stay, but worked my way into the hole again and down rung by rung till safely at the bottom, my heart pumping a little less with exertion than nervousness. Anyway I had done it!

When we returned to London, I was loth indeed to leave the ship and would gladly have sailed with her to Japan, but had to join my proper one for I had only been loaned to the P&O. It was now the realization came that I must give up, once and for all, the habit of clinging to the known and the past. And, facing the matter squarely, it ceased to be a trouble thereafter and I never looked back to any ship with regrets when it became necessary to leave one for another.

We sailed from London for Beira, our point of return, with one hundred and sixty passengers. Besides the dispensary where I saw first crew and then passengers each morning, there was a little hospital cabin with two beds, not bunks. I wondered what happened if one had a sick person from either sex. Did one put them together? I was to find out in due course.

As we cast off and moved out the first necessity was to overcome my shyness and try to make friends with the passengers. So whenever I saw one or two alone on the deck I went up to them and made a few trite overtures, introducing myself. Before sailing I had had a most useful tip. This was not to drink at the bar with them since it meant standing a round of expensive liqueurs probably, and quickly my payroll would decrease. If you wanted you could ask them to your cabin for a drink privately, and so need only entertain whom you liked. This proved itself invaluable for all my years at sea.

At dinner in the saloon I had a table of six to myself, each Senior Officer having to be host to some passengers. Never being much of a conversationalist, the meal began in silence and nothing was heard but the sipping of soup and the scrape of seven spoons against their plates. Racking my brains for something to start the ball rolling, all I could think of to say was: "Are you all seasoned travelers?" This produced a few nods except for one young woman who said shyly:

"No, this is my first voyage."

"Ah," I said genially, "mine too," intending to encourage her. But instead of being encouraged she looked at me aghast for a moment, and buried her head once more in her plate.

"You are the ship's doc, aren't you?" then asked a man at the end of the table.

"That's right," I replied, shuddering at the horrible abbreviation, an aversion to which I never overcame, like Prof. and Cap.

At once the young woman looked up with relief written all over her face: "Oh," she breathed, "I thought you were the Captain!" That broke the ice!

Rough seas did not affect me, and after we left the greyness of the Bay and entered the Mediterranean where water and sky were both blue, the excellent food, five course lunches, and seven course dinners were beginning to tell not only on the passengers but also on myself. Then I bethought me to hold P.T. classes daily after tea on the foredeck. This brought me into closer contact with the passengers than anything else could have. Perhaps some twenty responded to my invitation, and in swimming costume we met and began physical exercises followed by ball games with two huge medicine balls the Mate had made for me. These were amusement for spectators as well as players; even the bridge looked down through its binoculars to see the antics while less venturesome passengers lined the rail of the upper deck and shouted encouragement. Very quickly I became known to all, which no amount of chatting or drinking would have perfected. The one fear of all the passengers is the drunken surgeon and unfortunately there [are] all too many of them at sea where gin is six shillings a bottle — or was in those days. Many go to sea because they have already ruined their lives ashore in this manner, and on joining every ship I had to live down the reputation of the "gin-drinking ship's doc." I also volunteered to look after the children in the swimming pool in the afternoons, thus giving parents a much needed rest and allowing me to be legitimately out of uniform while teaching the younger ones how to swim.

Port Said was my first view of the East where exotic goods could be bought at equally exotic prices and where noise and dust were part of normal life. And from then on the East exerted its lure. I would lean on the rail as we went through the Suez Canal and watch the land so close by with its extending desert and camels ambling up the stretch of road, which lined the canal, taking no notice of the jeeps that whizzed by them. Port Sudan produced vultures perched on housetops in revolting fashion, and the Fuzzy-Wuzzies who were the dockworkers there, their uncut hair matted with camel dung to give it a nice "set." And then there was Aden, with its brown and barren mountains and RAF station, all so hot and dusty.

The heat in the Red Sea was appalling and there was much work to do. One old lady of 75, traveling alone had a hemorrhage from a duodenal ulcer and then became *non compos mentis*. She thought she was at home, and her fellow cabin-mates protested against her activities so I put her into the hospital. Then one evening a middle-aged man jumped off a hatch cover out of sheer joie-de-vivre and managed to break his fibula. Pain and the heat of his cabin, which he shared with three others, caused him to ask to be put in the hospital. So I found out the answer to the question that had first puzzled me — and in they went together!

At Mombasa where the majority disembarked, this man invited me up to Nairobi for a weekend, and, having the Captain's permission, I flew up. My only companion in the small aeroplane, incredibly, turned out to be someone from Folkestone also. Although I did not know him, he even lived on the same road as we had, but further down the town. At Nairobi I was taken to see the Great Rift Valley and the National Reserve Park, where the animals wander freely and you can watch from a car as lions come and rub themselves against the mudguards. But if you get out it is the last thing you ever do.

The Captain was friendly for he had approved of my P.T. experiment, being something of a physical fitness enthusiast himself. He was also somewhat eccentric and his cabin was a veritable arsenal. On the bulkheads were a bow and three iron tipped arrows, an African panga, or curved knife, a Japanese samurai sword, and a naval sword, the latter a relic of his midshipman days, since he had been called up for the Great War. In one corner of his cabin stood an airgun and sporting gun, and in another a lion rifle. Sometimes he would amuse himself at sea shooting the cushions with the bow and arrow, he would shoot at shite-hawks with the airgun when at anchor. He, the Chief Engineer and myself all carried bicycles and the trio could be seen going ashore together and then deviating according to tastes; the former two to the nearest golf course and myself to explore the countryside. The carrying of a bicycle was the means of my seeing far more than most officers ever saw of their ports of call, coupled with the fact that I had more time off in port since I did not have to work cargo or overhaul engines. I cycled in Mombasa, Dar es Salaam, and Tanga and also in the Portuguese colonies of Lourenco Marques, Beira, and Mozambique Island when we went there on the second trip.

One thing was very noticeable about the native populations of the two colonies. In the Portuguese there was never a raggedly dressed negro. They had their own townlets with properly built houses and roads laid out at right angles running through them. There were no restrictions on their going to any café or hotel if they wished but, as they were mostly workers, they had not the means for the better class places. In short there was no obvious color bar enforced. On the other hand the dockworkers were speeded on in their work by a foreman wielding a rope's end. In the British colonies, in contrast, there were no overt acts of violence. But the majority of negroes were ragged and lived in shacks with thatched tops, put down anywhere there might be a space for them outside the town. Their standard of living was incomparably lower. But which was the happier, who can say?

To one to whom Tarzan had been a youthful hero Africa was sadly disappointing, for where was the jungle? All about was scrub, no trees of any considerable size. The Africa of my dreams vanished abruptly!

Most of the passengers left the ship at Mombasa with only a few going on further. For the return the majority would embark again there. Meanwhile there was little for me to do, and I joined the classes the Third Mate was holding for the Lifeboat Ticket. It is desirable that as many of the ship's company as possible hold this Ticket since, in the event of having to abandon ship, there is more chance of one person with some knowledge being in charge of each lifeboat. We had to know: how to lower it, its construction, its stores and the rations allowable daily, the distress signals, the names of all parts of the boat and sails, and how to row and sail it. Also we had to know how to box the compass to sixty-four points. The Indian crew had to take the exam in English and to understand all orders thus. And so we spent many a pleasant time out in the harbor, taking in turns to cox and row.

One afternoon when he had no work to do, the Third suggested taking a lifeboat over to explore one of the many Arab dhows that lay around us.* These plied from Mombasa to the Persian Gulf, often carrying, if rumor was to be believed, slaves as cargo. So he and I, one apprentice and the Second Purser rowed over, and without asking permission first, climbed up the rope ladder that hung over the side onto the deck.

The dhow's Mate appeared, a villainous looking specimen with a squint and two broken front teeth, attired in an ankle-length dirty white shirt, but he showed no surprise or animosity. Instead he led us aft where apparently the Captain's quarters were, for on the poop was a ledge running round covered with thick rugs and cushions on which we sat crossed legged. The Captain, he told the Third, who seemed to be able to understand him in a version of Hindi, was ashore but we must have some refreshment. And he clapped his hands, in storybook style, and a negro brought coffee, thick and black in tiny cups and a plate of brown sticky sweetmeat of which we had to partake for the sake of good manners. There was a chronometer compass and a log-line, the former made in England, and this was all their navigational apparatus. We explored the whole ship; it would take only deck cargo, which was already laded and consisted of bales upon bales of hemp. Only the galley was below deck and there, looking down through

* A dhow is a kind of sailing boat traditionally used in the Indian Ocean and the Red Sea. They have lateen sails which are triangular and are mounted in a slanted fashion.

the small hatch we saw the negro cook, probably a slave, sitting puffing away at an enormous hookah. At once the Third dropped down beside him and taking the hookah tried his hand at it too. He was a youngster who believed in having as much experience of everything as possible, even hookahs and dhows.

She was well kept and spotlessly clean, the decks having been holystoned to make them almost white, and there was new paintwork round the gunwale, for some of the dhows are very ornate. Astern on both sides was a little box-like projection, also heavily painted outside, the starboard one more so than the port, and these according to the third were the "heads," the ornate one for the Captain and the other for the rest of the crew. A hole in the bottom of each box made a flush system quite superfluous. Finally we inspected the eye on either side of the bows, since the habit of giving boats eyes to see where they are going seems to date back to pre-civilization period, and is world wide.

The return voyage was uneventful with under a hundred passengers. I took to playing shove ha'penny each night after dinner with the Chief at a shilling a game, but when I was ten shillings up he decided he had had enough and found some other source of amusement.

Back in London the Lifeboat Ticket examination was held almost immediately. The theory was easy and then each candidate in turn had to take the examination out in the boat and bring it alongside anywhere he wanted, while the rest formed the crew. In the heat of the test it was inevitable that I suddenly reverted to river terms, telling the crew to "Easy!" (instead of "ship oars") with the result that we rammed the wall. However the examiner understood what had happened and gave me a second chance, and I managed to bring her alongside neatly. My oral test and the lowering of the boat had been satisfactory, so I passed and had the fact stamped in my Discharge Book to my pride.

The second voyage was to be the last this ship would ever do for she was thirty two years old and on her return would go to the scrapyard. As if to prove that there was life in her yet, we acquired a new passenger when half way down the Red Sea, one that the agents knew nothing of. This was a premature baby, only twenty-seven weeks in uterine, and no one knew that the mother was even pregnant for she was a bigly made woman and hardly showed. One day she sat down on a deck chair, which gave way under her. The fall started her bleeding and labor pains began. Of all this I was in blissful ignorance until six o'clock one morning when the stewardess called me saying there had been a woman in labor all night and would I please see her.

"Nonsense," I replied sleepily, "there are none such on board." But finally convinced I had a look and found it all too true. The baby was there, in good position and very much alive. I put her into the hospital cabin thinking it might be a false alarm but by after breakfast the head had gone down, which meant things were going to happen.

That morning I was not on the Captain's inspection round, instead I was trying to make the mite breathe which it only consented to do after being plunged into the hot water that inevitably appeared. It was 13 inches long and weighed three and a quarter pounds on the butcher's scales, and it was a boy! Great was the excitement among the passengers when they heard of it for the stewardess spread the story quickly, and the women downed their deck quilts and picked up knitting needles and set about knitting for the little stranger, unaware of its minute size, with the result that a pair of blue bootees made it two little caps!

The mother had no difficulty and hardly lost any blood. On the third evening I brought her into dinner in the saloon and had a seat put for her at my table. As she came in a round of applause greeted her from the passengers. I had not expected that the baby would live being so premature, but it defied textbook lore and thrived, probably the heat of the Red Sea being responsible and I had to put up daily bulletins of its progress. The Captain christened it in champagne, and on the great sports day every passenger ship holds, a silver beer mug was presented to it along with a little sailor doll with the name of the ship on its hat.

We left Beira for the last time flying the paying-off pennant to signify the ship's last voyage. The Third Mate had been busy sewing it on the way out, and it was ninety-six feet long, three feet for every year of the ship's life. The first yard carried the company's flag, with St. Patrick's cross on white ground. All the ships in port hooted thrice their farewell for it is a sad occasion when a ship is doomed, and whenever we came into port or left, the same greetings would be accorded us.

We sailed up the English Channel on a Sunday morning and for the first time I passed Folkestone from the sea, seeing clearly well known landmarks like the Grand and Metropole Hotels and Trinity Church. We had only been away three months but a wave of nostalgia swept over me, and I wondered how the sailors of old felt coming up the channel after years at sea.

First we had to unload on the continent, and I did a tour of Hamburg with the Chief Engineer, by a special tour bus. The conductor who described the sights had a sense of humor. He would point to ruin after ruin and say "that was bombed by the British" and when we passed a fine upstanding redbrick building he said mournfully, "That is the Income Tax Department. That was NOT bombed by the British!"

Then to Scotland to the breakers! In London everything had been taken off the ship that was movable except what was in the cabins and needed for the saloon. On the last morning in Scotland, there was a rush to acquire what was going. Two sweating kalassies carried the stout Purser's biggest tin trunk down the gangway stuffed with food. The Chief had rolls of carpets from his cabin, and I had five pounds of beef and nearly as many of butter I intended taking to the aunts. Also, I took possession of a set of B.I. wine glasses, which had been in my cabin; for, we were told, what we did not take the breakers would. The glasses were a valued souvenir for some time to come.

This leave was a longish one; I had to wait for a ship. And it was now that I took the step which ultimately led to my discovery, for I called on the editor of Debrett with my birth certificate and asked that the entry in his annual edition be changed to the correct names, since in this only was there any remnant of my past surviving. He was kindness itself and acknowledged my claim to the baronetcy if I survived my brother who, although he had married during the war or shortly afterwards, had no children. He also promised that any alteration made in Debrett would automatically be followed in Burke's *Peerage*. That this was eventually unfulfilled, led to a discrepancy between the two books that at long last someone noticed. However that was still in the future. I had several happy years as a perfectly ordinary human being in the eyes of the world, yet to come.

Needless to say Bobby was very angry when he learned of it, for of all things he feared especially was publicity in this connection, quite wrongly gauging the reactions of his friends in the matter.

After a while I was offered the *Dunera*, a troopship that was to sail for Japan and bring back the "Glorious Glosters" from Korea who were now in Kobe.* On this ship formality was almost Royal Navy. If one went to speak to the Captain one was supposed to salute, not merely just first thing in the morning as had previously been the custom on my other ships. There was a C.O. and a skeleton army staff as part of the company to look after the ex-prisoners on the way home and we also took back to Singapore the coronation contingent of the Gurkhas, including the fabulous Major Perna Lei, the only non-British officer to hold the king's commission and who

---

* The "Glorious Glosters" were a highly decorated infantry regiment of the British Army.

was also a V.C.* He was much addicted to playing deck quoits and it was hard to believe he was the martinet that stories made him out to be. We also had sundry other officers returning from leave in the Far East, any of whom had been over for the coronation too.

It was a colorful scene in the saloon at dinner with all the varied mess kits. The Army has trouser stripe and cummerbund to match, red, purple, yellow, green or what have you, the tight trousers and shiny jack boots were also in evidence; there were a few naval officers who were dressed as we were, some Royal Air Force and Women's Auxiliary Air Force and a dozen of Queen Alexandra's Nurses in their own bright red and grey attire. The Gurkas we put ashore in Singapore and a full-kilted bagpipe band met them, marching up and down on the quayside while they disembarked. It was on this occasion that I made the acquaintance of my French cousin who lived in Singapore and thereafter, whenever I was on a ship that called there, he gave me the best hospitality and made my shore-leave most enjoyable.

But from there we began to hear rumors of trouble on board the *Asturias*, the ship which fetched the first batch of ex-prisoners. There were stories of beatings-up and how one man had been pushed overboard and when rescued had been pushed overboard again. And the ship had nearly been set on fire. The Captain, who was a Chief-Officer-acting-Captain, and the C.O. became frankly nervous as we plowed on towards Japan. At each port we had fresh news along the same lines.

At last we reached Kobe, and I was seeing Japan for the first time. We lay opposite H.M.S. *Ocean*, the aircraft carrier, and I was invited to lunch in the officers' mess and shown over the ship by the young Surgeon Lieutenant. We had some days to wait and one afternoon I went with Sparks to Hiroshima by bus. We looked for signs of damage and could find none. It had been totally rebuilt and on modern lines. Any English blitzed city showed itself infinitely worse.

Another day we went to an opera in Kyoto given by a famous all-women troupe who therefore had to take men's parts. And here I also saw my first Buddhist temple, knowing nothing about that religion then, and I did not find it in the least inspiring.

Then came the day for embarking the troops. Many seemed oddly reluctant to be going home, and at the last minute a police van came down

---

* The Gurkhas were a Nepalese British Army regiment sent to Singapore (then a colony of the British Empire) to celebrate Queen Elizabeth II's coronation.

to the wharf and three soldiers were forced out struggling and pushed up the gangway. Two at last reached the top, but the third fought the M.P.'s so hard that at last he was bundled back into the van and driven off.

One would have expected they would all have been longing to go home. It was the chaplain who explained to me what had happened over a beer in my cabin one evening. It was the usual well-meaning War Office muddle. Some old blimp had said: "Bring the dear boys down to Kobe and give them all the money they want from their back pay and let them have a good time." And of course the inevitable happened. The Japanese prostitutes moved out promptly and took up quarters in or near Hiroshima and up went their prices. And since venereal disease is almost universal in Japan, the soldiers lost all their money and syphilis was of epidemic proportions among them. So many of them did not know how to meet their families again. A little wisdom and restraint might have saved much suffering.

As soon as we sailed, there were threats publicly made of beating up those who had informed on their companions while in prison camps. And soon there were several cases of men in the ship's hospital with battered features and other damage. Fortunately no one was pushed overboard, but one soldier was found in the lavatory with his throat cut down to the larynx. He lived for only twenty minutes after being discovered and could not speak. The body was brought home in the refrigerator since there were certain anomalous signs about it. But naturally a verdict of suicide was brought in since it suited the politicians to have these men treated as heroes. Their progress as heroes, moreover, was reported in the press, and as they read about themselves in the newspapers we bought in Aden and Port Said, they became even more undisciplined, answering back to their officers and showing them not even the barest respect. Finally, some of them demanded to the Chief Officer that they be treated as civilians since their term of service had long since expired, hence they should no longer be subject to military discipline. On an inspiration he agreed at once, saying that of course their pay would stop from that day in consequence. No more was heard of their being civilians.

It was with relief that we docked in Southampton without the ship having suffered any serious damage. I left it gladly for trooping was not my line, and set about looking for a passenger ship again. But the B.I. had only twelve passengers to offer, for all but one of her M class ships had been scrapped, and she had only two large liners.

Perhaps another company might have something better to offer. If I stayed on I would all too quickly forget my medicine, not being an old hand like some of the surgeons who had taken to the sea after retiring. At length I signed a contract with the China Navigation Company of which I knew nothing, and found myself at London Airport with a ticket to Hong Kong, a five days flight in those days and in company with two ex apprentices, one from the P&O and a Third Mate. We were to be out for four years and the chief job of the company was to take Moslem Pilgrims from Singapore and Penang to Jeddah for Mecca for the Haj, or annual pilgrimage, which every Moslem is supposed to make once in his lifetime. There would be plenty of work to do, of that I was assured.

CHAPTER 9

On the Haj

Before leaving London a visit to Charing Cross Road bookshops had produced every possible book written about Gurdjieff and Ouspensky, including Nicoll's *Psychological Commentaries* which were to prove the most valuable of them all. As yet only the first three volumes were out, later to be superseded by the fourth, but they gave ample food for thought. Unfortunately they had to come by sea with my trunk, as air luggage was limited so that, when I was to need them most, they still had not arrived.

The need arose due to my being kept in Hong Kong for five weeks. Knowing no one, with Christmas just ahead, I developed an acute sense of loneliness and frustration. Mostly it was my own fault. I was at first promised a ship that was on contract to the B.I. sailing between Hong Kong and Calcutta, which tickled my fancy very much, having just left the B.I. She would be carrying passengers, which meant a chance of making a little extra, but the only other surgeon in the fleet demanded it as his right so at the last moment we were switched. The result was that I was filled with resentment and, as my Captain was to put it later, when we had become good friends, I was "just a pain in the neck." Hence he made no friendly overtures as he might otherwise have done. Nor were the other officers the sort I was accustomed to, for the best do not care to sign on four-year contracts, and several had left other companies for various reasons. There was none of the formality and etiquette to which the B.I. had accustomed me, and no one to whom I could talk.

I mooned round Hong Kong, becoming more and more discontented and depressed the nearer Christmas came. And Hong Kong itself is noted for its aloofness to strangers. The Mission to Seamen padre happened to be ill and even there there was nothing to be found. Then one morning just before Christmas I was wandering disconsolately round the cathedral grounds, kicking stones, when a young clergyman hurried by, of the type that had "keen Christian" written all over him. In desperation for someone to talk to I made some trite remark, and while obviously in haste, he stopped. The next moment I was pouring out all the story of my loneliness to him. At once he asked me over to Kowloon where his vicarage was, to have supper with him and his wife. She was Oxford and he had been Cambridge so we would have much in common. And then I was invited to stay there on Christmas Eve and as they had two small children, all the ingredients were there for a good Christmas.

This is worth recording because, when my luggage came, and I began to read Nicoll's books, there was the condition stated clearly how self-pity augments any negative emotion. I had certainly been in an acute state of self-pity, and therein one could read how to tackle it. From then on, through better understanding, it became possible to cope with a negative state. Although often this meant a prolonged struggle, because, as Gurdjieff says, we love our negative emotions, and indulge in a kind of mental masochism, tormenting ourselves by living over and over again unhappy or embarrassing events to the extent of keeping ourselves awake at night with them. How much energy is wasted thereby and illness caused is unknown!

At last the ship's repairs were finished and we sailed first for Japan and then to Indonesia, where, so the Mate told me, deck officers who were wise locked themselves into their cabins while the cargo was unloading. This was because, since the Communist regime, the dockers would think nothing of slashing a bale of cloth and taking out a piece before throwing the rest down. Three European Mates had lost their lives trying to interfere, as was their duty, one being gutted with a boathook, and now they left it to the insurance companies to stand the loss.

The river up to the Palembang was all I imagined the Amazon might be, brown and turbid, lined with jungle, dense and matted, and the air was sticky and hot. While in port there was nothing but a native type village about which sand blew in great profusion. Still, Indonesia was a new country to me, and every new country was an experience. Here we were to pick up some hundred or so Chinese adolescents who had been promised by the fatherly Communist regime of Red China that they would be given free higher education. All had bought bicycles in the hopes of selling them at a good profit ashore but, from the stories that trickled through to Hong Kong, all their hopes were dashed on arrival in their home land, where their bicycles were confiscated and they were drafted into the Army, men and women alike, and saw no higher education but only indoctrination. But this news had not yet filtered through as far as Indonesia.

With March we stopped our cargo carrying and headed for Singapore, which would be our headquarters for the Haj, the great pilgrimage to Mecca. Annually shipping companies are on contract to ferry pilgrims back and forth and we could take between 1,100 and 1,200 Malayans, filling the holds with this human cargo. A hospital was erected across the hatch covers on the well deck to hold some thirty beds, women on one side, men on the other, for on the return many would be starving, dying of vitamin deficiency and with various diseases. Once their money was finished the Arabs had no further use for them and they could lie sick and neglected. Such hospitals as were provided, we heard, were staffed either by local or Indian doctors and the notorious custom of selling drugs was rife so that, even if admitted, the patients said they were given no more than a bed.

Two surgeons were required per ship for this and I was given a Junior Assistant who turned out to be far senior to me medically, being an M.R.C.P. M.R.C.S. But he had had a stroke and was doing a sea-trip because he could no longer practice ashore and had officially retired. His brain had been affected and he had lost all powers of concentration so that he could no longer follow the thread of a conversation in the saloon for more than a minute before he lost it. He would be quite incapable of learning any Malayan or finding out a case history. It transpired that his method was to give every patient a purgative first time and if he came again not cured then to see what was wrong with him. We had successive surgeries and the Portugo-Malay Dresser, who was an old hand at this game, used to keep back any people he thought were really ill for my surgery in the evening.

About half joined the ship in Singapore and the rest in Penang, that most beautiful island of the East. Having not brought my bicycle I bought an old one cheap here, and then, one day, cycled round the whole island, forty six miles, in circumference. In the furthest away corner, riding along a narrow track through jungle, I came upon a prehistoric monster about twenty yards away in the act of crossing the road. It had a tiny head, lizard like, longish neck, fat cylindrical body and a tremendous tail, and was covered in mud-brown scales. It gave one look at me as I got off and tried to come nearer quietly without frightening it, so as to be able to take a photograph, but then it did a sudden about turn and disappeared into the undergrowth. All I saw as I reached the spot was a final flick of the great tail. Inquiries elicited the information that it was probably a monitor lizard, about six feet long; although they were rare on the island, there were plenty of them on the mainland of Kedah just opposite.

Three trips we had to make to Jeddah before the Feast of Ramadan would end the month of fasting, during which no Moslem will eat between sunrise and sunset or even drink water, although dockworkers were allowed to suck ice on the grounds of it being neither food nor drink. Then we would have to lie in Aden for three weeks before we could collect the pilgrims and transport them back again. There would be a week in Singapore probably each time and a few days in Penang on the trip back.

The first two voyages were relatively uneventful. Minor operations, seasickness and trivial diseases were the general routine. They were all supposed to have been passed as fit to travel by a shore doctor before being allowed on board, but in the East this amounts to a little palm greasing. On the second day out an old man informed me he had not passed urine for six days, please would I do something. On examination he was found to have advanced cancer of the prostate and not even the smallest catheter would pass, so there was nothing for it but to insert a supra-pubic tube through the abdominal wall under a local anesthetic and relieve the bladder. Five days later, though the operation was successful, the patient died of a heart attack. It is not a moment for mourning by Moslems when they are on the Haj, for if they die at any point while making the pilgrimage they go straight to the arms of Allah. We carried a big white-painted coffin-box and after the body had been washed and dressed, it was put in the box and the engines were stopped. When the weigh was off the ship this was slung out over the stern from a small davit rigged especially for the purpose, and it was lowered to the water level. Then the box was tipped and the body slid into the sea.

When we arrived in Jeddah for the first time the agent was waiting. He rushed up to the Captain to tell him to warn the crew on no account to take a cigarette ashore with them. A few days before a seaman off an Italian ship lying astern of us had stopped in the street to light a cigarette. At once he had been pounced on by the police, and been given twenty strokes on the spot for smoking in public between sunrise and sunset during the Feast of Ramadan!

Nor was any alcohol to be shown on deck; stewards might not carry their trays in view of the wharf. And he added another story. An American cabin boy on his first voyage had heard of a friend on another ship at the same wharf. He had therefore taken a couple of bottles of beer down as a present to him. The port police had arrested him the moment he was off the gangway and by the time the agents got him out of jail, his ship had had to sail without him. Jeddah was definitely not a port for tourists!

I went ashore that evening, full of curiosity, in company with the half Arab, half Malay Second Steward, who knew the ropes and I had my camera concealed under a coat. The light was going but I managed to get a few photographs of the town. Perhaps the most impressive thing about it was that when the trumpet blew for prayers, the many moneychangers left their tables with the piles of gold and silver coin unguarded and went to the appointed place. But then theft was punished by amputation of the hand and failure to attend prayers by severe flogging. At six o'clock they eat and smoke after a twelve hour fast, and everywhere in the cafés men would be sitting round the tables heaped with food and waiting until the trumpet should allow them to help themselves.

Running back empty there was no work to do. The crew was Chinese and unlike the Indians they are not malingerers; if a Chinese sailor came to the surgery, I could be quite certain he was really ill. It was then I asked the Old Man if I could teach the Lifeboat Ticket classes which were really the Third Mate's duty. But our Third was often too busy with his private business when off the bridge to find time for the classes, and I had nothing to do all day. He agreed when he learned I had my Ticket recently, and so daily Chinese would come up and settle on the poop deck around the surgery and learn, from pictures drawn on the deck or door in chalk, the names of the equipment and parts of boat and sail. They knew no word of English but they, too, would have to take the exam in English. By dint of solid repetition they learned the orders for lowering the boat, rowing, the boxing of the compass, and the names of the equipment. And now I began to wonder why all three types of foodstuffs for shipwrecked sailors should be those which normally one cannot eat without washing them down with fluid, since water is the main problem in a lifeboat at sea. There was tinned condensed milk, barley sugar and the driest of dry biscuits. This was the normal peacetime provender and the fishing lines that had been furnished during the war had been removed again immediately after. Why? One could not help wondering.

In Penang and again in Singapore we went out for practice in rowing and sailing. When the day of the exam arrived my class passed, thirteen out of thirteen. The examiner confided to the Old Man afterwards, that it was the first time he had ever heard a Chinese at the tiller shouting "In . . . Out"! But he also added that he had never seen a lifeboat crew keep better time—as the result of my employing river-racing methods!

On the second voyage out we had an unusual excitement. I was sitting making a rug along with the Captain, for we had bought one between us and each started at opposite ends, when the Second came full speed across the deck to say "Man overboard!" Up leapt the Captain up the iron ladder three steps at a time, and I ran up on deck to see what was happening. A Blue Funnel Line ship was passing close to us even as our engines stopped, and we swung to port while the O flag, signifying "man overboard" was run up to the masthead. Immediately the Blue Funnel ship also stopped her engines and veered away to her portside. Together we circled the area for more than an hour but there was nothing to be seen.

I learned the story from my Dresser whose English was excellent. One of the passengers, a middle-aged man, had been taken on the Haj by his wife and other relatives because for some time past he had behaved oddly. On board he had caused a little trouble among the passengers, sometimes going up to one or another and pushing him off a seat and sitting on it himself. Once I had been asked to see him but there were no grounds found for putting him under restraint. This evening, it seemed, he had been talking to some of his friends on deck when he had seen this Blue Funnel ship bearing down quite close to us and going in the opposite direction.

"I'm going back to Singapore on that ship," he had said and had gone below, collected his dispatch case and all his wife's jewelry and returned on deck. Before anyone realized what he intended he had climbed over the rail and dropped into the sea. As he had not jumped clear he must have been sucked into the propellers immediately and so no trace of him was found. His wife was very annoyed about her jewelry, we heard!

On our return to Singapore I did a day trip by plane to Sarawark to see that far famed colony, although one could not see much in the short time allowed. As I could find nowhere for lunch, I contented myself with a cup of tea and a cake but good feeding on board ship had made me too confident. For many years after the war I had always carried glucose to ensure staving off any hypoglycemic attack, the specter of which always haunted me and I had many narrow shaves. Now I had been ten hours without proper food. Feeling a bit odd, I took a taxi down to the wharf where a launch would take me back to the ship, since in Singapore we had to anchor outside the reef. I got out of the taxi and next thing I knew, two hours later, I was in the Singapore hospital with a lump like a tennis ball on my head and a long scalp wound. There I remained till the day we sailed when the Dresser was sent to fetch me down, of which I remember nothing.

But with 1,100 odd pilgrims I could not stay long in my bunk. Next day I forced myself up and to the surgery, for the old doctor could not look after the patients alone. Convalescence only prolongs an illness; I had long since decided that as the result of much experience. At the garage there had been no opportunity for convalescing, nor was there now.

There was good news waiting us in Jeddah for instead of having to lie in baking, dusty Aden for three weeks, we learned that our Aden agents had a cargo of rice for us to take to the Seychelles, Mahé Island, later to become famous for being the place of exile of Archbishop Makarios. This was a very lucky break for me for seldom did a ship go there, at least not one carrying an English surgeon. And here we saw the products of intermarriage between French, negroes and other Europeans, with the strangest conglomeration of racial characteristics. Two brothers ran the launch that took us ashore. One had dark straight hair, brown eyes and thin Western features, the other red hair, blue eyes and a grossly Negroid nose and mouth with prognathic jaw.

Ashore we saw the giant tortoises, relics of what the pirates found when they first discovered the uses of these islands as bases of refuge three hundred years ago. For there was no animal life then, only crocodiles and these tortoises, no poisonous insects or snakes, and they noted, as have all sailors since, the famous palm trees, differentiated as to sex into male and female palms, the nature of whose fruit had led General Gordon (later to die at Khartoum) to write a letter to the Royal Society to say that he believed he had discovered the original Garden of Eden. For here was the Tree of the Knowledge of Good and Evil! The letter was preserved in the island's museum.

It used to be thought that the Seychelles were the tops of the mountains of an ancient continent stretching from Africa to Malaya, but an ardent shell collector there, who supplied museums all over the world, told me he had found fossils and marine shells on the tops of the mountain which formed the center of the island. With him I had tea and he showed me his collection. Hence it must be surmised that the islands must have arisen out of the sea and possibly the land between Madagascar and India had subsided slowly again thereafter. For how else would anyone account for the presence of crocodiles, which are not noted as being marine animals and could hardly swim the thousand miles from Madagascar?

Mahé preserved its atmosphere of being a pirate island well. When we first sighted it, anchored on a sheet of blue water which had no ripple to disturb its surface, was the *Dolinda*, a three-masted schooner owned by an ex–Royal Naval Commander, who made regular trips to Madagascar taking any passengers who preferred real sea life to that of a floating hotel. Ashore the first sign presenting itself was that of The Pirates Arms, but one was hardly prepared for seeing at one of the tables in its dining room, a little old lady in flowered frock and big straw hat, who might have stepped out of any Kensington restaurant. This, my companion, the Indian port doctor, told me was the last surviving suffragette who had retired here for economic reasons, although quite unnecessarily. Her home was no more than a native shack on the beach.

The Club threw open its doors to the officers, delighted at having visitors. And this must be the only place in the whole world, outside its country of manufacture, where Irish whiskey takes predominance over all other drinks. The whole shelf in the Club was filled with it and it could be had in every house. It was in the Club that I met a man from Lincoln College, Oxford, and he took me back to his home on the mountain for supper while we reminisced over that "golden Oxford afternoon" we had both experienced. And here no one urged a friend to have one for the road, for the only flat metaled roadway ran for a mile along the beach through the town. For the rest, it had been bulldozed out of the mountainside, with hairpin bends and drops of hundreds of feet if you misjudged and no railing to give you any confidence. Some years later I was to have a similar ride among Ladakhi Mountains.

We left after three days much refreshed by our trip, and returned to Jeddah for the first batch of pilgrims going home again. The agent came on board and had dinner and a couple of drinks with the Mate in the secrecy of his cabin, since only when a ship came in did he get an opportunity of a drink in Southern Arabia. Then he offered to take some of the officers into town in his Land Rover.

As I heard the story subsequently, when called out of my bunk to treat the injured, the Rover had been swerving along the mile-long road that lay between docks and town, and then it had toppled over the bank that sloped to the shore and rolled into the sea. The back door had been flung open and the old doctor and the Third Mate had been thrown out. The Chief Engineer, two juniors and the agent climbed out through the front windows. The Chief then saw the old doctor lying at the bottom of the shallow water and held his head up until pain in his own back forced him to let go. Somehow he was dragged ashore and a passing taxi was persuaded, not without great difficulty, for the Arabs loathe supposedly drunken sailors coming to their teetotal shores, to take them back to the ship.

When I first saw them the surgeon was unconscious still, and the Chief was in severe pain and I suspected a lumbar fracture which would have to be x-rayed. Leaving the doctor to my Dresser we took the taxi out again to find a hospital and after some searching, for although there were hospitals, they would not admit us, we finally found a private nursing home whose owner consented to do the x-ray and confirmed the diagnosis. The first lumbar vertebra had been fractured.

It was two o'clock in the morning when I plastered him with a jacket on the after deck, stretched out between two trestle tables, and with the Malay Dresser and Mate assisting, and then went to look at my Junior Assistant. There was slight grazing down his bald scalp but no sign of any external contusion and he was now asleep breathing quietly. In fact, he remained asleep for the entire voyage back and accused the Captain and myself of conspiring to starve him since he never remembered having his meals, going to sleep again immediately after. The rest escaped with grazings and bruises except the Third who had been caught by the door handle on his privates. A hematoma of the scrotum resulted and there were inevitable nautical jokes at his expense when I gave him a pad and bandage to wear to protect his clothes from the ooze!

Up all night, the next morning we took on nearly twelve hundred pilgrims with many cases requiring to be put in the hospital straightaway. One youth with pneumonia had been lying on a concrete floor for a couple of weeks, and anyone who knows what bedsores are like from a soft bed can have some idea of what his body was like, made raw from contact with the hard floor. Another was a woman with gross edema, her hands and arms more swollen than her legs and feet, which is unusual. She was too far gone with Vitamin B deficiency to survive and died within twenty-four hours. It was a busy voyage back, no time for rug making or anything else except the evening game of deck quoits the Captain insisted on after tea every day. He was an adept and I won only two or three times during the whole time I was on that ship, but it gave him some exercise and me a little recreation.

This time it was the outward voyages which were dull and empty. But on one the agents gave us an Arab man, his two wives and thirteen children. They had demanded from him a deposit lest he was refused permission to land as sometimes happened and then they would have had to carry him back free. He had refused to pay it but a friend guaranteed him to the company. Then when we reached Jeddah there was an envoy from the King of Saudi Arabia to meet him on the quayside with a welcoming letter from

His Highness, for it seemed he was a highly esteemed merchant who was well known in Royal circles!

At this time I had been trying to work in the manner prescribed by Gurdjieff in respect of self knowledge and self awareness, and, indeed, there was plenty of scope, for I did not get on well with my brother officers, and my only friend on board was the Captain who was in the same situation, although he had many friends ashore in Hong Kong and Singapore. Once one realizes when one is in the process of being anxious, worried, becoming angry or being irritated, then one can check it and alter the course of events. It is when one only realizes it afterwards that nothing can be done. And the more one gets to know oneself the sooner one spots oneself in the middle of a reaction, and in time one can spot it as it arises and then it can be prevented altogether. Finally that type of reaction, too often checked, ceases to arise at all and one has mastered it. But it does not happen overnight; it takes months or even years but gradually a change takes place. This is the essence of the Gurdjieffian teaching and the aspect of it on which Ouspensky in particular concentrated. And Nicoll's whole three volumes were devoted to it.

We came down to Singapore for the last time and the special hospital was dismantled, the extra Malay crew and my Dresser discharged, also the old doctor who was now just getting up a little. And then we went on to Hong Kong.

I was not happy with the company after this first year, and with aid from the Captain I persuaded it to give me my discharge. Instead of repatriating me to England I asked to give me a berth to Australia in one of their ships running there, for it had two large passenger ships from Sydney to Hong Kong and Japan. Finally it was agreed that I should travel up to Japan with the ship and then transfer in January to one going to Sydney. The purpose behind my desire to visit Australia was to see this aunt, our mother's sister, with whom I had been having more frequent correspondence since first going to sea. She always expressed the hope that I might one day come to her. She had of course been informed of the change and accepted it without comment.

We sailed for Japan in December and after the heat of Arabia and Singapore the cold was striking. Powdered snow lay over the wharf at Yokohama, after heavy frost in Osaka and Nagasaki. Here we were to spend Christmas and on the Eve I went with the Old Man on the short train ride to Tokyo where we amused ourselves in the biggest store, Selfridge in type, finding our way to the toy department where we played with trains till it was time to go for tea.

That evening a party was given by the agents on the ship and Japanese waitresses were imported, clad in their kimonos. They not only served drinks but danced with the officers, and dancing with a Japanese girl is an experience never to be forgotten! One of my partners was intrigued with my beard since they do not grow on Japanese men and she stood on tiptoe to touch it, to my acute embarrassment. Then she beckoned to another waitress to come over and feel it too; meanwhile I had to suffer ribald comments of the Captain and the officers who were greatly amused.

New Year's Eve we spent in Kobe and it was to be [my] last night on the ship about which I was not sorry, although I was sorry to be leaving my friendly Captain. Later, when on leave, he came to visit me when I was working in Oxford, out of curiosity to see that wonderful place he had heard so much about. I took him out in a punt on the river and we recalled Lifeboat Ticket days. Together we went to The King's Arms in Kobe, an exact replica of an Olde Englishe Pubbe, built by an enterprising Englishman. It had oaken beams, a public bar with darts board, private bar and dining room with sporting prints round the wall. It was a home from home to many an exiled Englishman. At midnight drinks were on the house in traditional style, and then two young B.I. officers came in and started throwing Chinese crackers and the party broke up. It was a good finish to a period in which I had learned a great deal but the usefulness of which was exhausted.

When I reached Sydney there was Aunt Mary waiting for me, stout and short and attired in blue coat and skirt and a large blue hat. We were equally shy of this meeting and could think of nothing to say after the pecking kiss we exchanged. Then she took me home to her lodgings.

The rest of my five weeks stay in Australia was devoted to finding her somewhere decent to live. With a curious streak of snobbery she had a single room in a decrepit house situated, however, in the best residential area of Sydney. But the landlord cared nothing for its internal state and the wallpaper was hanging off the walls of her long, thin room and all water had to be fetched from the landing below. In one room she cooked, washed, slept and entertained. But she had only a small pension, and although it appeared I had many Australian cousins none of them helped her. Things being what they were I was not prepared to meet any of these relatives and have to explain things to them all. So I concentrated on trying to find new quarters for Aunt Mary, which was impeded by the stream of snobbery making her refuse places in any but the best locality that were beyond my pocket. At last it turned out she owned a plot of land in Adelaide and wanted to build a house on it. So finally I subscribed substantially to this project, and on a later voyage was to see the result. Meanwhile I tried to elicit information concerning our mother but she seemed to have forgotten much, being then seventy-five years old.

Her chief interest was in man-made effects and she wanted to take me touring Sydney to show me buildings and parks rather than the works of nature, like the Blue Mountains, of which I did not hear until a day or so before leaving and so failed to see. But we did go to Botany Bay and La Perouse in a river steamer, to see where Captain Cooke landed. On this trip came a sister of that Dublin Zoology Professor who had been kind to me when I was a medical student, and who had given me a letter to her when I went to sea in case I should ever go to Sydney. She was good company but unfortunately Aunt Mary became jealous of her, since she was younger than herself and more active.

At first I thought to get a job working my passage home on some ship but I did not know till afterwards that palm-greasing was involved here also and, despite my M.N. Discharge Book, I could not find a vacancy. Eventually, irked by Sydney accents and crudity I bought a berth in one of the emigrant ships returning to England, staffed by German crew and at tourist prices. There was every nationality on board, educated and uneducated, and to wile away the voyage we formed a "university" having classes in various languages and lectures on philosophy from myself which became more popular than one would have expected from the subject matter.

But the highlights of the voyage were the call at Naples and seeing the Pyramids of Egypt. Naples I now visited for the first time respectably dressed, instead of in shorts and tee shirt, and although there was no time to go and see Pompeii again as I would have liked, for the place fascinated me, I went to the museum in Naples where so many of the Pompeian relics were housed. Impressed on my memory is a gladiator's helmet, green from copper oxide, embossed with every possible scene of violence of which man is capable, doubtless to stimulate the cruel side of its owner's nature who had to live by violence or else die from it.

The Pyramids were indeed a lucky break since as surgeon I could never have left the ship at Suez and gone by land to Port Said. But Cooks Tours had laid on cars and guides for the passengers and we were in Cairo in the morning after leaving at dawn. It seemed it was possible to visit the Pyramids by tram, which upset all my preconceived notions of them being alone in the desert. Actually the tram line ends about half a mile from them and then you hire a horse or a camel to finish the journey. Despite big notices that no tipping was allowed, the animal owners wait until their victim is mounted and walking along a rocky path and then demand to know how much you will give them. If you refused they will beat your mount with a stick and force it into a canter if a horse and a run if a camel and terrified at all the rocks below you, you will probably capitulate. This game was tried on every member of my party, and only those who could ride well remained adamant.

The Sphinx affected me greatly, much more so than the sight of the Pyramids. There was something about the calm imperturbability of its battered features which had been a target for the Mameluke's firing practice, that made me want to sit and contemplate them. But flies and ragged urchins and sellers of all sorts of bric-a-brac prevented this effectually. If one wanted to, one would have to go by night and probably modern commercialism would even then make it impossible.

When we reached Southampton I had been away a year and a half, the longest ever away from England and it was April, the best time of the year to be at home. May morning would see me in Oxford to celebrate my birthday and I would not rush after another job for a couple of months at least. Also I had in mind to take my old garage friend G. on a cycle trip in Italy if he could get a fortnight's holiday and his wife would let him go.

CHAPTER 10

Round the World

First I went to Folkestone to see that Toto and Daisy were all right and to pay my respects to Mr. Whyte, as at every visit. He was growing very old now, a change was apparent each time I saw him and he could no longer read his beloved books all day or follow the argumentations of the modern philosophers, so he said. Twenty-two years had passed since I had first gone shyly to his rooms to learn Latin, and now he lived a lonely life in lodgings where the landlady was kind to him. He would still be seen out in the town on mornings in his duffle coat, but walking now with a stick and no longer striding along as had been his wont.

And Toto and Daisy, they were sitting crouched over a wisp of smoke when I arrived one chilly night after supper. Only one lump of coal might be put on the fire at a time and there were bricks on each side to keep it small. Their toes were out of their slippers and their dressing gowns ragged. What could one do with them? This fiction of poverty led the inhabitants who had known Bob and me as children to ask why something was not done by us for our aunts in their old age when they had looked after us in our youth. Of course nobody recognized me these days with my beard, and they thought I had gone off and deserted my family.

It would be useless buying them dressing gowns; they would refuse to wear them. "What's the good when there is no one to see us?" Toto would say as she had said so many times. Next morning I went out and bought them both a pair of moccasins, fur trimmed. Perhaps they might be persuaded to wear those. And each day I would take Daisy out to lunch in the town; poor Daisy, half-starving while paying amply for her keep. Toto would refuse to go: "I don't want you to spend your money on me." Only on my last day could she be inveigled.

If I brought them butter it would be mixed with margarine and eked out until it had gone bad; only by lavishly buttering Daisy's bread myself could she have a real taste of it. Once when chocolate had been in short supply in England I had brought two big chocolate Easter eggs from Dublin. Years later I found them, still intact, but now pale and anemic from old age. They had been too pretty to break and eat—so put them away and forget all about them! They had no servant. They could not afford one, and though I offered to pay the wages for a woman to live in, the offer was refused. "We prefer it like this." Toto always used the royal "we" without giving Daisy a chance to offer her opinion. Poor Toto! She was like a shriveled up walnut in its shell, and when she died but a couple of years later she left a sum in the realm of £24,000! I often wondered what had made her so; early habit caught from her own mother certainly had had its effect, for Granny was the same. But chiefly lack of self-observation, awareness of what was going on so mechanically inside her seemed to be the main cause—the cause of all psychopathies and neuroses.

From Folkestone I went to Bristol to my friend the Canon and we celebrated the night of my return, as always, with dinner at the Royal Hotel and topped up the kitty, one-tenth of my pay-off, and he would tell me of cases which had been helped, over a cigar and an Irish whiskey in the lounge. To him also I could tell all my deepest feelings about things and he never laughed or scoffed but was always understanding.

Then on to G. who by now was working in the Post Office and living in a prefab house. I found his six-year-old son at an elementary school in a class in which he was the only one who could read, since his father had taught him before he ever went to school. G. had also once bought the boy a comic at Woolworths on the theme of the *Iliad* and so enthralled with it had the boy been that all the children in the housing estate had been marshaled into Greeks and Trojans for the purpose of pitched battles to the annoyance of their parents who demanded of G. why he wanted to fill his child's head with that nonsense.

That the boy should be wasting his time in an elementary school seemed absurd when he appeared to have a good brain and potentiality. I looked through the telephone book for preparatory schools and hit on the one nearest to their home. After my talking to the Headmaster and guaranteeing the fees, G. and young G. went for an interview. There the lad got himself admitted! The Head gave him a short story to read and then questioned him about it.

"Where did the fox go at night?" he asked.

"To his lair," answered little G.

"No, no," said the Head, "that's not what it says in the book. Now think, where did it go?"

Young G. was puzzled but once again said definitely, "To its lair."

The Head showed him the book. "There you are," he said, "you see it says it went to its den."

G. gave him a withering look and said in a voice full of scorn, "A den is a lair!"

The Head nodded with a grin at his father and said, "The boy's in."

There was the uniform to be provided and I paid the fees for a year ahead explaining that I might be at sea when the time came round again but not to worry, as soon as I returned I would settle up annually, and promised G. if the boy could win a scholarship I would see him through public school as well. But some effort must come from him himself, for his own sake.

And thus I tried to repay G. for his faithfulness to me during those garage days. He himself had always longed to go to a proper school and now he would relive his own schooldays in his son's. Eventually the boy did win a scholarship and showed himself worthy of the experiment, but that was not until his Uncle Michael had disappeared in India, and would see him no more.

After May Morning in Oxford at which I managed to get both my tutor and his wife up before dawn, I thought to do the Merchant Navy Defense Training as the rail and dock strike were on and there were no ships moving. This idea sprung from Gurdjieffian reading wherein it advocated new avenues of action, the newer and stranger the better, to open up latent centers, especially if an effort was required to do it. And embarking on something quite unknown was always an effort to me.

I stayed at the Mission to Seamen, Victoria Dock Road, whose acquaintance I had already made and of which I can never speak too highly. I got to know it well in due course but this was the first time I had put up there, having only been in for meals or cinema shows before. And now in the evenings I would serve in the canteen and on Sunday nights I joined the country dancing and found it far more enjoyable than the ballroom variety. Every morning I went into Westminster where the training ship H.M.S. *Chrysanthemum* was lying. Because of the rail strike only a few were attending that session: a Blue Funnel apprentice, a P&O cadet, a middle-aged Third Mate who had returned to sea after becoming fed up with married life, three seamen and myself. Lectures were held by a Naval Commander who became properly embarrassed when he discovered he had to lecture on first aid and survival at sea to a doctor! We also had practical classes under a C.P.O. in manning and firing the light anti-aircraft guns fitted to merchant ships in war-time. And on the final passing out test, because there were so few of us, we were running round in circles with sixty pound shells in our arms—into the gun, one man pretended to fire, out again, and back on the rack, and then take another . . . it was good exercise! Now another stamp would be put in my Discharge Book when I next signed on articles; the only surgeon to have that one, I believe.

Before the course was ended I had become accepted by Ellerman Lines but they had said that they would have no ship until three weeks after the dock strike would have ended, since they were all lying idle in Liverpool. So I notified G. of an intended cycling holiday in Italy, would he like to come? He would! And we met in Folkestone and stayed the night with the aunts before crossing to France. As before I started from Naples and showed him Pompeii, which impressed him as much as it had me, and then to Rome which thrilled him, since he had been improving his classical knowledge with library books, thinking now to educate himself so as to be some use to his son and not to let him down in later years.

One night we camped by Lake Trasimene, and went to sleep on hay damp from a thunderstorm, hoping to dream of the Roman legions which were routed there by Hannibal, and to hear the tramp of marching feet, but all that happened was that we got colds and mine turned to laryngitis so that by the time we reached Florence, for which I was primed with information about the Medici in general and Lorenzo the Magnificent in particular, I could only whisper and that painfully. It was not until Pisa that my voice returned, in time to explain Galileo's famous experiment from the Leaning Tower.

We ended our trip at Nice and returned by train to Folkestone and on the very next day a telegram came from Ellerman's asking me to fly to New York and join the *City of Johannesburg*, whose surgeon had been put ashore. Here was an adventure indeed! There was a romantic sound about it. Moreover she was on a round-the-world voyage, although it would take longer than eighty days! And we would visit Red China from which she had come with cargo for Canada, already unloaded, chiefly human hair and pigs' bristles!

New York was disappointing, but only what might have been expected, all size, and money and shouting about both. We went through the Panama Canal and up to Los Angeles where, because the ship had been to Red China, the most absurd precautions were taken. Armed sailors were put on board with a Geiger counter while in the sling; despite the fact we had completely unloaded the Chinese cargo in Canada. And when we took on a few passengers, missionaries going to Manila, their luggage was also tested. Great was the excitement when over one missionary's trunk the needle swung up. He was made to unpack it all and there, at the bottom, was an alarm clock with a phosphorescent dial!

It was on this ship I that had my first initiation into deck work. After Hong Kong we had no passengers, for none might go to China, and there was no work to do, so one morning I helped the Second Mate take to pieces the electric sounding machine which he wanted painted, chipping off the old paintwork first. And for the first time I handled a chipping hammer. Ere long I was to become an enthusiastic chipper and painter. There was something very satisfying about hitting a bar and having a large bit of paint and rust fly off. The Captain, though not friendly, raised no objection and the Mate taught me how not to leave "holidays" or little specks unpainted. Next I checked the lifeboat equipment with the Third who was a Belfast man and knew of my doctor friends there. It is pleasant sitting up in a lifeboat under the sun in only a pair of shorts; idly checking this and that, making sure none of the food has been stolen and exchanging notes of home. And he taught me how to splice and fix eyes and toggles.

Tien-Tsin was our first sight of Red China; an ex-German seaside resort, it had all the atmosphere of decadence, although from the sea it looked very like a continental town with church spires and Teutonic architecture. But ashore one saw the churches were barbwired off, their windows broken, large houses turned into tenement flats and an awful uniformity about everybody. There was only one costume, white shirt and royal blue cotton trousers, for men and women alike. Here and there one saw a face that betokened breeding but afraid to show it.

Up the Yangtze River we went for about 250 miles to enter Shanghai. Here all binoculars, telescopes, cameras, sextants and the like were put under seal and also all the distress signals from the lifeboats, though what the *raison d'être* of that could be is hard to know so far inland. We were allowed to go ashore but must stay in the middle of the town; if we wandered outside we would be put in prison. A car would fetch us to the Seamen's Club and give us a run round the city at night, so we were told.

Shanghai had not lost all its prosperous look although all foreign bank buildings had been turned into tenements, but the goods in the shops were shoddy and the roads and houses were in need of repair. The Seamen's Club was solely for propaganda purposes. There one could buy the best Chinese goods at reduced prices, including the brocades which were so popular with one's womenfolk at home, China tea of the green leaf variety, and pictures painted on silk. Here I bethought me of the matron and nurses at my Dublin hospital to whom brocade dress lengths would be something beyond belief, but incredibly cheap for me. I bought four lengths for four of them and posted them back with a note for the customs stating that it was an unsolicited and quite unexpected gift from an ex-R.M.O. and the added appeal: "Be kind!" The Irish Customs wrote underneath: "Noted" and let them in free, which shows that officialdom everywhere is not devoid of humanity.

But one afternoon going ashore on foot we had to pass through dockland on the way to the town. There we saw the real Red China. Human beings were used to haul the carts of cargo loads to the docks, two pushing and two pulling. On the way was a hump-back bridge and they were almost on all fours pulling their loads over that. One of these hauliers was a woman about six months pregnant, and I wished I had a camera to show the Reddened West what Communism in China really was like. But that was why the cameras had all been impounded: to keep its spectacles rose tinted. On the table in the Club were all sorts of free magazines displaying the great achievements of China, which could be taken away, and there also were copies of the *Daily Worker* from England . . .

Coming down to Hong Kong we ran into my first typhoon. Admittedly it was only a little one but still, a typhoon. It began one evening and after we had gone to bed the ship began to heave and bucket and seemed sometimes to be standing on her nose and then again on her stern. After some hours of this there was a sudden deathly calm: we had reached the middle of the typhoon. This lasted about half an hour when we began to come out the other side and the bucketing started again. There was no sleep to be had that night since one could not stay still in one's bunk nor even lying on the deck athwart ships, which was usually the solution to a rough sea, for she seemed to roll everyway. As a result we did not call at Hong Kong again, but went down outside the island to Ceylon since India was omitted from our itinerary, too many other ships from the fleet serving her.

We had been out five and a half months when we returned to London and I went first to Folkestone because, during the voyage, I had had a letter to say Toto had had a fall and broken her femur and was in hospital. Then Daisy had written a graphic description of how she had found Toto lying on the kitchen floor and could not lift her up, and Bobby wrote more caustically to say that on his arrival from Ireland at the hospital he had found they thought she was a pauper and he had had to go out and buy her some respectable nightdresses. But by now she had left hospital, her bone pinned, and they had abandoned the house and gone to live in rooms on Earl Avenue, where I found Daisy looking much fatter and better, being now reasonably well fed, and Toto walking with a stick quite briskly. She was then 87 and Daisy was 83.

If the furniture was left in the house they would have to go on paying rates so it was agreed that I should clear it out, and sell what was not wanted since house and furniture was willed to me anyway. I started with the loft under the roof. It was full of long, flat dress boxes crammed to capacity with paper bags and there were rows of empty jam jars on the floor. Not a bag, not a jar had been thrown away since we had been there, it seemed! At the crucial moment [a] Bob-A-Job scout rang the doorbell and was welcomed in and given 2/6 at the end of a strenuous afternoon's work that ended with his taking all the jars away whither he would.

When I reached Toto's room and opened the long box ottoman, there on the top were the moccasins I had bought less than a year before, re-wrapped in their tissue paper, too good to use. Beneath were boxes on boxes of notepapers from Christmas and birthday presents, excellent pre-War quality, some of it with our crest on, but Toto had always insisted on buying a Woolworth pad, thus spending money unnecessarily, rather than use "good" stuff. Further down was a child's fancy dress I had worn once, made of raffia, a red flannel petticoat of a quality never seen these days, and two pairs of striped flannel drawers, minus their seat, that must have belonged to her during the Victorian years. At this point I rang up the local Social Service and asked them to send a van to collect clothes suitable for old age pensioners of aged hospital patients!

Next I found the strip of cloth with my 22 Girl Guide badges on it, together with Guide tie, hat and belt—but there! It would take too long to list all the treasures that had been cherished for nearly a century, since they included a doll's tea set from Toto's own childhood. I collected everything useful to them, including the notepaper and the moccasins and packed two suitcases one for each, Daisy's filled chiefly with her photographs, framed or in albums. For myself I took my grandfather's sword and the paintings of our ancestors and the books. Finally, the furniture realized only £25, so old-fashioned was it. Then I was offered the *City of Bath* on the American-Indian run, due to sail for New York early in December carrying as passenger a relative of Sir John Ellerman.

This was the happiest ship I had known since my first, with a Captain who allowed everyone to do his job without interference, and a jovial Aberdonian Mate named Willie. The crossing took eight days from storms. One had to hold one's soup plate up to one's chin in order to take part at all. One day when I was sitting on the heavy settee large enough for four, with a thick-piled carpet between it and the deck, the whole thing slid across the lounge—which gives some indication of the list of the ship. I went out on deck holding on all the way, and the waves were breaking over the upper deck and drenching the bridge in spray. There was something impressive about a huge wave curling up in front of us, ready to dash itself to death on the foredeck. All around were grey mountains of water, foam crested, rising and falling in maddened motion. Yet I could never feel the justification for the adjective "cruel" so applied to the sea. Even though it swallowed you up it was friendly and gave you a final resting place in the quiet of its depths.*

Then we sailed for England and now began my real deck career with a willing Mate who said he could always do with an extra hand for chipping and painting. I worked with the apprentices and the carpenter, doing anything they did and when we were near Bombay the Fourth Mate went down with malaria. When I went to tell Willie he said half jokingly, "O.K., if you've put him to bed you'll have to come on the fo'c'sle head with me this afternoon when we enter port. Must have someone to shout through the megaphone."

This was too good a chance to miss. I decided to take him seriously and when the pilot was on board I presented myself to Willie on the fo'c'sle in my uniform complete with cap which I usually never wore.

He laughed and gave me the megaphone since this ship had no telephone system and told me to stand half way down the foredeck and repeat to the Bridge anything he said but, he added, not to repeat what was not intended for the Bridge! Now Willie had a strong Aberdonian accent and

* The following paragraph is then crossed out: "We spent Christmas in St. John's Halifax, a dismal day and the seamen's club closed because no one would attend to give them a party till Boxing Day. It was not the Flying Angel but a lay-run institute. At Victoria Dock Road in London Christmas was made as homely as possible for all seamen in port. A parcel for each, dinner games and dancing as well as a service in the chapel for those who wanted but never compulsory."

I had no knowledge of throwing out lines and typing up or casting off and did not know what he might be likely to say.

"Cable leaving us now," I sang out hopefully through the megaphone at one point and heard a faint echo of laughter from the Captain who signaled with his hand that he had understood that "Cable leaving astern" was meant! He did not mind; it was chiefly a formality anyway, just in case the bridge could not see whether a line was still fast or had been let go.

The Fourth was still ill when we left again, but this time going through the locks I had gathered more knowledge of what it was all about. And I looked after the cables on the port side while the Mate kept a weather-eye open but confined himself to the starboard side. On leaving we passed under the stern of the P&O ship the *Canton*, and an officer and passengers came aft to look at the odd phenomenon of an officer on the fo'c'sle and a surgeon bawling out orders at the kalassies heaving out lines. It definitely would *never* be done in the P&O!

Ashore in Bombay I cycled round one afternoon and came upon a fair sized café where I stopped for tea. Across the middle of the room slung from the ceiling was a long board with a text painted on it: "Speak not the sins of another while thou thyself art a sinner." And the name following was Baha'u'llah of which I had never heard. The manager, seeing my interest in this, came down with a couple of tracts on the Baha'i faith and told me something of it in English. The earth receives Teachers and Master Teachers in plenty but never recognizes them. Some it kills, others it merely laughs at or brings charges against. To none does it listen. The Teacher secures a group of followers and shortly after His death, or even before, His Teaching is distorted to suit the false values of mankind. In years even more recent than those of Baha'u'llah, who was executed at the end of the last century, Gurdjieff had suffered this, and was aware of it even before he died.

As we sailed up the Hooghly River for Calcutta, the temperature on the fo'c'sle head was registered as 125° and 112° on the bridge. Here tragedy overtook the ship. We lay for many days sweltering in the dock, and the Third Engineer, after imbibing a little too freely one night, complained next day of sickness but he was not very ill for he had been out on deck in the afternoon playing. I gave him some nausea-allaying medicine and thought no more of it. That night I was called up because he had been found unconscious under the shower. Heat stroke had set in. When I saw him he had been carried to his cabin but was delirious shouting and fighting everyone. I tried to force glucose-saline fluid down him, but he would not take it and spat it back at me. Nor could I take his temperature but he was burning hot. He must be got to hospital immediately.

It took two hours after telephoning the ambulance to come, two hours in which his life might have been saved. He was unconscious on arrival with a temperature at 109°. We put a drip up and poured water over his covering sheet and turned the fan full blast on him but to no avail. I stayed with him all night and in [the] early morning he died. From a happy ship friction set in, the heat and the effect on the other officers' nerves of this taking its toll. But I saw little of it. Two days later I went down with bacillary dysentery, probably caught off a kalassie I had put ashore with it in Bombay and had half carried up the steps of the hospital as he had become weak through constant motions.

The ship sailed away without me and I regretfully said "goodbye" to the Captain and Willie the Mate, although glad to be going home so unexpectedly early. Two weeks I remained and was supposedly cured. Then on my birthday I was given an air ticket for London while another of the company's ships would take my gear. Just before leaving all hell broke loose again, but I told no one for I wanted to get back to England out of the heat of Calcutta. But things were so bad on the plane and I could keep nothing down that the pilot radioed for an ambulance to meet the plane at Northolt, and I was taken to Greenwich Seamen's Hospital, for I had been traveling D.B.S. (i.e., as Distressed British Seaman) on my Seaman's Identity Card instead of a passport, according to international convention for such cases, and so the Seamen's hospital could not refuse me admission as other hospitals might.

I was there another two and a half weeks before really cured and, though still weak, went to Belfast to recuperate and finish something I had started during the happier days at sea. This was a small volume of poetry which was to be immodestly entitled *Poems of Truth* and consisted of twenty sets of verses with prose counterparts on what it said: Truth!

Only once before had I had a spell of versification and that was sonnet forms or epic narrative usually on subjects either religious or martial. But an abrupt end was put to it when one day an aunt asked me what I intended to be and I rashly said, "A poet!" She had given a loud laugh and said, "Don't be so silly, you haven't got it in you!" and from that moment I wrote no more until now.

The urge to write would come upon me as soon as I had awakened in the early morning and the poem would often be finished before breakfast. Not that it was automatic writing by any means since I had to count syllables and was often stuck for a rhyme, but on the whole it flowed easily and if I was interrupted I could pick up the threads again without trouble. Illness had affected the output, however, and the last three poems (not necessarily the last three in the book) were achieved only with difficulty.

Publishing poetry is quite impossible unless you are already recognized, and so I paid for its production and launched 1,000 copies on the unsuspecting public without, however, apparently making much impression. They were strongly Gurdjieffian in sentiment but I was not at home long enough to supervise distribution and only one shop took the stock when I went to sea again never to return. Incidentally the printer, incredibly, turned out to be the young brother of one of those three good school-friends of mine, and I had known him as a little boy! But I did not find this out until the typescript was in his hands.

It was during my leisurely convalescence, since there was no immediate hurry to recover this time that I was put in touch with one of the Ouspensky groups functioning in London. This was of great interest after all I had read of those who were "in the Work," and I went to the meetings eagerly. But try as I would I could not see that the Work ideas had really penetrated in more than one or two. "It is possible to know everything and to understand nothing," as Gurdjieff himself said.* One lady was definitely evolved above the average, and the leader of the group, an exceptionally kindly man, was on the threshold and watchful. But the rest seemed rather to be playing with ideas as things apart from themselves. They were also all agreed that no one could do any work on himself outside a Group, hence my couple of years of attempting this were of no avail, so they said. In fact although it is a strong point in the teaching that you need the Group, with companions who will help you to know yourself, and leaders who know how to bring out the best and the worst in you and create the right situation for you to master at the right moment, as Gurdjieff so often did with his pupils. Yet it is also the teaching of the Work that life itself is your Teacher. Of course a combination of the two is the best. To have the aid of the Group and then to go away and practice alone using the imitations and adversities of daily life for a while. But this they did not agree with. On the other hand to refuse the aid of a Group when one was available is equally wrong and stupid.

It was interesting to watch the different members both during the meetings and the social evenings afterwards. It was customary to adjourn to the local's private bar after a meeting and there they seemed so quickly to forget the Work idea of mindfulness, or self-awareness, and were lost in ordinary conversation and jokes as if they had never heard of it. After watching this on several occasions I asked one man who had been attending for some years, just to test a theory: "Do you use the pub also as a means of Work?"

* The last sentence was added by hand.

His beer glass paused en route to his mouth and he looked at me in astonishment. "I suppose we do," he said slowly, so obviously meaning they did not, which was the impression I had had from it all.

One man there, a typical Edwardian type of English gentleman, was really a sincere striver, doing his best to apply everything he learned to his life but he was hampered by a not over good brain. But in his persistent efforts at self conquest, although not understanding cosmology or the deeper theories, he surpassed all those who could beat him intellectually. They seemed all to be badly impeded by the clichés of the Work idea of their being "in It," and therefore something apart from all those who were not.

When fit again I was assigned to *The City of Oxford* (a name which tickled my fancy) loading in Hull and sailing for South Africa from which she would sail to Australia. I introduced myself to the Mate and his apprentice. He was one of the nicest fellows anyone could hope to meet and his pet abomination was being called Jacky, so he saw at once my own hatred of the term "doc" which I never managed to overcome and which earned me a reputation for uncertain temper; since a Junior Officer addressing me thus almost inevitably received a frozen look and curt response. However, to most of my friends on all ships I was just "Mike."

On the way out I had a cable to say Toto had died of strangulated femora hernia and Bobby was taking Daisy over to Ireland to live with him. At last she would have peace from nagging and good living!

We sailed down to South Africa with a few passengers, about half a dozen, and Table Mountain was completely concealed from view under a low cloud as we passed Cape Town. The Mate had given me the whole of the fo'c'sle to myself to chip and paint, a job that would take many weeks alone, and it was very pleasant working up there under a not too hot sun with a gentle swell, away from everybody and only in shorts. One lady passenger voiced the opinion of others one day by saying, "It's so nice to see you working, then we know you will not be drunk if anyone need you suddenly!"

We were in Durban a week and there saw the color bar in action for the first time. But there was one place where it could not be exerted, as a result of its constitution, and that was in the Mission to Seamen, and on filmshow night negroes, Indians, Chinese and Europeans, all Seamen sat together. May it long continue! It was the Mission which organized an outing on a Sunday to the valley of a Thousand Hills, where an enterprising café owner employs a Zulu family to do war dances for his clients, in return for hut accommodation and what they can make from the audiences. They were wearing nothing but raffia skirts and bracelets and the day was cold and drizzly, so that the completely naked children sat huddled at the doors of their huts with noses that might have been blue had they not been chocolate.

From Durban we sailed for Port Pirie in ballast and encountered the Roaring Forties. One week from Australia there was the job of shoveling overboard the sand to enable the ship's draught to be reduced for the depth of the harbor. With the Mate, the serang (or Indian bo'sun) and the kalassies we shoveled all day for six days but shortly what might have been a boring task became a treasure hunt, for the dockers in Durban, purloining goods, had hidden some of them in our sand, hoping for an opportunity of recovering them before we sailed. Bales of cotton cloth, of good worsted, carpentry tools and what-not, we dug up in turn. The Mate, knowing when the Nelson touch should be applied, left it in the hands of the serang whose perquisites they were, to keep what he wanted and sell the rest cheap to the crew. But it made the game exciting, for you never knew what your shovel would hit next.

Port Pirie is a one-horse-and-buggy town, if ever there was one, and down the High Street trundles the railway engine on its lines. I did read sometime later in a newspaper that it had been blown away in a cyclone, but not as to whether it has been replaced or not. From there we went to Adelaide, and there to see Aunt Mary once again, now in her new house, but with hardly a stick of furniture, it seemed, and with a nice back garden which she was too old to dig. Assistance was needed!

Now I had made quite a close friend on board of the Fourth Engineer who had come up to my cabin one day and inquired if I knew Latin, if so would I teach him as he wanted to leave the sea and become a doctor and he had been trying to work with a *Teach Yourself* book, not very successfully. Thereafter he came up every evening before surgery and after the lesson he would sit and rant against humanity. He appeared to have been disillusioned in respect of all religions and philosophies of which he had read a surprising amount.

It was amusing in that I could recapture some of my old argumentative skill which had grown rusty while chipping paint, but at the same time Dennis was looking for something although as yet he was immersed in his frustration and self pity at not having found anything.

We covered all the usual ground again and again and then one night I thought to give him a typescript of Ouspensky's lectures on negative emotion which I had bought at the last meeting I had been to in London.

At ten o'clock that night when I was lying on my bunk reading the door of the cabin burst open and in precipitated the Fourth unceremoniously, waving the typescript.

"This is IT, Mike," he cried, loud enough to wake the Second Mate next door. "This is what I have been looking for. Who is this man and what else has he written?"

I smiled at this enthusiasm and signed to him to come in and be a bit more quiet since the Second would be on watch from twelve to four in the morning. Then I had to tell him all I knew about Gurdjieff and Ouspensky, which was not very much and finally lent him Nicoll's fourth volume, which had since come out and which could stand alone and contained everything anyone could want for a lifetime of Working.

The friendship grew thereafter and he and I spent all our spare time at Aunt Mary's house, digging up the field behind and sowing vegetables for her to eke out her diet. He was of invaluable assistance.

But what were these ideas that had struck him and myself so forcibly, him even more violently than me, since he had reached a greater depth of despair?

"Man is not one but many." We are all a multiplicity of little selves and not a single individuality as we imagine. Our job is to eradicate these and to form a real Self. This I was to find later was Buddhist doctrine.

"Your being attracts your life." You suffer what you suffer because you are what you are. And the more one thinks about this the truer it appears, although at first sight we tend to blame circumstances, especially upbringing and heredity. But Gurdjieff had something to say about that too.

"People tend to complain about their lives and imagine if only things had been different, if they had had better education or social status or more money, they would have been different, and better." But, "the circumstances in which you were born are the best for you to work upon. They are the very things that give you Force if you work against them." (And I might well claim the right to know the Truth of that one!)

Then came one that had struck me most forcibly.

"Ideally speaking, however terrible the event that life can create for you, you should be able not to identify with it, not to put yourself in its power." And again, "Nothing in life can hurt you if only you learn not to re-act." And again, "Something unpleasant happens to you. Logically you have every right to be upset. But if you are it is solely your own fault. You do not *have* to be negative."

And from this follows the corollary:

"Understand clearly that we cannot change the events but only our way of taking them, we cannot reform the world, we can only reform ourselves."

"Whatever the circumstances, if you take them as Work, you will come out unbroken."

Again, too, Gurdjieff stressed the mechanicalness of man which he does not realize and will not admit, thinking he is awake and conscious in life whereas he is a mere robot, a puppet of forces of which he has no inkling, simply because he is asleep.

"We re-act: we do not act. We are mechanical, not conscious. The Work as well as all esoteric Teachings says emphatically that Man is asleep and he must try to awaken from that state of sleep. Anyone who lives and dies in a state of sleep has completely failed to realize what is the most important thing in Life to strive for."

Herein I had found the answer to my childhood question: What is the purpose of Life in general and of my life in particular? The answer is, "to evolve spiritually. To develop and to cease to be a slave to all those little selves, our moods and desires, which hold us enthralled." Hitherto I had been ever-ready to reform others, now I saw this was impossible. It is oneself that makes others behave towards one as they do. It is one's job to become impervious to all the unpleasantness of life, if one can and to consider others. And this is a major task of gigantic proportions. I had already found that if one had seemingly ceased to be resentful about some things that had angered one before, if once one gave way to a negative emotion on a large scale, all one's old selves rushed back in again immediately and had once more to be eradicated, though being weaker this was easier than the first time.

Now the written word can appeal to the Reason. On an intellectual basis this has appealed to many. But to be effective it must also appeal to the Emotions. Unless it appeals to both, then it has no effect on our Being. "It is only when you apply the Work Ideas to yourself that the Work can change you."

I was to learn much later that this was also the keynote of Tibetan Buddhism, for throughout the Tibetan canon there is constantly recurring the warning that the knowledge attained must be applied to behavior: this is the famous Union of Wisdom and Method, symbolized in the Bell and Dorje in the hands of Dorje Chung.

In my own *Poems of Truth*, in one of the short prose accompaniments to a poem I had entitled "Knowing and Being" I had said, "Truth may be likened to a ladder that stretches from Heaven to Earth. Its rungs are the rungs of Being, its sides are the sides of Knowledge, and the act of climbing it is Understanding. Even as a ladder is no longer a ladder if sides or rungs are removed, and even as we are unable to climb it unless our hands grip the sides and our feet are planted firmly on the rungs, so also there is no

Knowledge obtainable without improvement in the level of Being, nor can any such improvement come without access to further Knowledge."

As yet unaware of Tibetan Buddhism, it had appeared a self-evident Truth when I first read of how Work Ideas must be applied, first and foremost. Those who are interested in the intellectual side of Gurdjieffianism, the abstruse cosmology, are in the majority, and in failing to grasp the very basic principle they only succeed in adding another little "I" to all those already there, instead of excluding any, the "I" of intellectual pride.

But one has to be dissatisfied with oneself and with Life first.

"If we really feel we are all wrong we begin to change," and

"The meaning of the Work is to change the way you think," and

"If a man would work on himself instead of praying to a far-off God to save the people, he would find the Kingdom of Heaven is not indifferent to those who try."

Again, Gurdjieff had stressed the comfortable false picture we each of us have of ourselves, while we scout as quite untrue the accurate picture others have of us. This went home the deepest in me. "It is astonishingly terrifying that one can go on for years living with a false picture of oneself and even with a wish to know, yet to have no real picture of how one manifests oneself to others."

The Buddha put the first fetter by which men are bound as Self-delusion. So long as that remains we can do nothing, make no progress because we imagine we are progressing and really are not. But it was Gurdjieff who offered a practical way of dispelling this illusion.

"Self-observation may bring home to you what everybody else knows about you and has criticized, perhaps to your face, which previously only had the effect of infuriating you." And he had given the most valuable of all tips, namely, when someone criticizes you, instead of immediately reacting in protest with counter-charges or excuses ("you do not understand me," or "Well, you're another") say nothing but go home quietly and think about it. Is this true, that he says of me? And ninety-nine times out of a hundred, even a hundred times, one will have to admit that it is, if we are honest. Then one can start to work on it, for one will recognize its appearance in ourselves next time that which was criticized arises.

If we want to know how we look in a new suit, whether it fits or not, we do not trust to our own judgment, looking down at ourselves or even in the mirror; almost certainly we go along and ask someone else how we look in it. Yet concerning our mental clothing we think we ourselves are the best judge; that we know ourselves better than others know us, who can see us from the outside. If someone tells us some act or emotion of ours is ugly or does not become us, at once we are angry and try to retaliate and then comfort ourselves with renewed assurance that all we are is perfect or if not quite perfect there are excellent reasons why we are as we are.

From the first time I read this I made a resolve never to defend myself against such criticism again nor to counter-abuse, but to listen and then think and for this piece of advice in the Gurdjieff-Ouspensky books I can never be too grateful. Then one can begin to view objectively the question: why does so-and-so not like me? And the odds are on discovering that one had ridden rough shod over his feelings at some time. So one gets to know oneself a little.

And the better one knows oneself the better one can understand other people, seeing oneself very often mirrored in them. So one can guess why one does this or another behaves like that, for we can associate their quaint conduct with episodes in our own lives. And understanding is the basis of Compassion, as also Compassion is of Understanding.

These then are the basic ideas at the root of the Work, culled from various sources which can be obtained by any who are searching and have not yet met them. But Gurdjieff, in his life time was condemned as a witch-doctor in France, as a libertine in England, as a decadent in India, as a "gluttonous man and a wine-bibber," but of Someone else that was also said . . . Those who seek may find; the rest will continue in their blissful mechanicalness, dead while living.

On the way to Fremantle the Mate told me he had reserved a treat for me: to go over the bows and paint the ship's crest which was the coat-of-arms of the *City of Oxford*, the red ox on the blue and silver striped ford. This was normally an apprentice's job.

When we were moored alongside, one morning the kalassies slung a stage over the prow and lashed it. The serang tested the lashings so that he should not have my blood on his head and then paint pots and brushes were lowered on to the stage by a line, and a kalassie slid down a rope to disengage them. I was about to follow with very mixed feelings about all this, exciting in anticipation as it had been, when the serang stopped me and heaved over a short rope ladder. This was a sop to my lack of experience as a sailor.

Once on the stage, what looked so easy from ashore, since I had seen sailors painting the outside of the ship many times from stages, proved difficult in the extreme; there was a light breeze and the stage swung back and forth and did not feel at all safe. I sat down, trying to look at my ease while brown faces peered down grinning. By wedging one foot against the bow I could keep it fairly still until the leg got tired. However I was determined not to give in and gradually first the ford and the ox was given a new coat. In the middle an apprentice put his head over and shouted that a man had had his leg crushed against the bulkhead by a crate. Not loth to leave my precarious perch I swarmed up the ladder and went to investigate the casualty—which one stitch sufficed in the end: the "crush" bringing something of an exaggeration, he having only suffered a small cut and bruising.

Now to return would be a great effort, for by no means would I admit to the Mate that I was scared stiff, fifty feet above the muddy river water of the dock. And in the end I finished it to his satisfaction, as he surveyed it from below.

We were now to sail for home via the Suez canal, a long stretch at sea, and I took the opportunity of acquiring the only remaining certificate that in my position I could get: the Steering certificate. This was usually done by deck hands hoping to secure a job as Quartermaster in due course. It required ten hours at the wheel and I set about, with the Captain's blessing, the two hour trick in the afternoon, under the eye of the Second Mate whose watch it was. This line, although it had Indian crews, carried English Quartermasters, who were nothing loth to be relieved and be able to sit outside the wheelhouse and have a smoke while I wrestled with the wheel.

Let no one imagine it is like a car which runs straight when the wheel is left alone. Every wave and current veers the bows and the whole time one must be turning a little to starboard and a little to port. Two points error either side is considered fair steering, mine were nearer five points, doubtless adding to the length of the day's run in consequence! Maximum concentration was required, the slightest woolgathering and one would find the compass needle awry. I had already done a little on the *Bath* on the way to India but had not had time to manage the full quota before going sick. But by the time we reached the Gulf of Aden I had my certificate with sixteen hours and could take a trick when I felt like it—provided the sea was not too rough, or we were not in confined areas.

The first thought of every seaman nearing port is of mail. Let those remember who have kin at sea. It is the same as with the hospital patient. Once in Rooksdown an officer had burst into tears when, on the tenth successive day, the Sister had to tell him there were no letters for him. And no one else laughed for we all might have done the same under similar circumstances.

So after three weeks at sea we were looking forward to our mail when Sparks brought a message to the Old Man. We were to anchor in the gulf and await further orders. The Suez crisis was on! We had of course heard about it from our wireless sets and had wondered what would be the position of the officers if we found ourselves at war with Nasser, since the crew was mainly Mahommedan. For a night and a day we lay at anchor and then we were ordered to sail via the Cape and put in at Lourenco Marques where it was promised our mail would await us. Apart from Chips who professed Communism we were behind Eden to a man and even thought of sending him a cable to that effect. As it turned out he could have done with all the moral support he could get.*

So away we sailed, leaving nautical oaths behind us wafting on breezes back to Aden. But the mail actually was awaiting us when nearly three weeks later we reached Lourenco Marques after six weeks at sea. This is an unusually long time for modern vessels unless they are cable ships. A sister-ship on the America-India run, diverted from Bombay, was less lucky and her mail had not arrived, the company would have to sail on to the States via the Cape with no news from home.

Rounding the Cape the weather was all it has ever been said to be by sailing ships and in number two hold the cargo of bags of grain shifted. There were sacks all over the deck and this, naturally, will alter the stability of the ship. So I spent a whole day with Chips hammering nails into planks, heaving bags into place and shoring them up, until once more all was ship-shape and Bristol fashion!

I enjoyed this deck work and was never happier than when there was a specific job to be done such as this. My seaman's jersey was by now plentifully bedaubed with paint and greases and my nails were broken and most un-surgeon-like. But it was a much better life than reading all the morning until the bar opened and then propping it up till lunch-time; sleeping off the effects of the meal and then having a quiet game of quoits or tennis till the bar re-opened, which was the more normal routine.

But this voyage I had a growing feeling that this life would soon end, that chipping and painting and manual work had served its purpose and soon would come a change. When I first went to sea I knew there would come a time when I should have to leave it again, when its use would be exhausted, and then the next door would be opened for me, since all else was subservient to this Search for Truth. I was still being pushed along by I knew not what and my medical career seemed primarily for the purpose of my seeing the world. It was never an end in itself.

* The last two sentences are handwritten additions.

CHAPTER 11

Interlude Ashore

As there was no call to go to Folkestone now I went first to Oxford via London where, as always, I called on Sir Harold Gillies at the London Clinic. He always seemed glad to see me and invariably reiterated that he was delighted he had undertaken my surgery since it had been so worthwhile. There were many who would not have and my debt to him can never be repaid. He died the year I went to Rizong, shortly after my return from there, and my Belfast doctor friends sent me the obituary notice from the *British Medical Journal.** His one aim had always been to make life tolerable for those who either Nature or man had ill-treated without regard to conventional views and to many a one he must have given renewed hope and a new start.

While at Oxford I realized an ambition that had been with me for some time past, that of visiting the DeLaWarr Laboratories of which I had heard much on and off. The "Black Box" or Diagnostic Instrument was not un-

---

* In the right margin there is a note: "check—1959 or 1960?" Then, directly above the word "Rizong" Dillon supplies the date "1960."

known to me since that obsessed young Scottish doctor had had one and I had been given ample proof of its efficiency even before we had taken it to pieces to see what made it work, and were little the wiser afterwards.

Throughout my sea career this Box and the subject of Radiesthesia, as the technique of its use is called, had been thrown up at me in the most unlikely places. One B.I. Second Mate had suddenly asked me one day: "Do you know anything about Radiesthesia?" I countered the question by one asking how he came to have heard the word at all. He told me a B.I. Captain was very interested in it and had talked about it often when they had been on the Bridge together. Again I heard it mentioned in Hong Kong but forget in what connection, and in India there are a number of practitioners working it.

So I found my way to the Laboratories and met Mr. DeLaWarr who showed me all around and expatiated on the wonderful things that might be discovered in the next few years there. The showmanship was superb and the whole layout was directed towards impressing the visitor.

Before the end of the afternoon at the Laboratories I had been offered a job there but I had already accepted a temporary post as casualty officer at a hospital near the docks in London and would have to do that first. Then I promised I would return for a while and work there, although the sea was still calling. But Oxford called the louder!

This hospital was to be my first experience of nationalized medicine which I had always been against in theory and now I was shocked at what I found. It seemed I was expected to give penicillin and anti-tetanus injections for every scratch, cut or graze that came in and not one penicillin but daily for five days, since the theory was that one would merely create an immunity. No wonder the Health Service costs had rocketed! Besides it was against my medical conscience to do this. Penicillin should only be used for spreading infection or prophylactically for a very dirty cut and anti-tetanus could be dangerous in itself. I had had a case in Dublin which had nearly collapsed and died as a result of an allergic reaction and I was loth to use it routinely. But, I was told, it must be this way these days and the courts did not seem to be aware of a distinction between an honest medical opinion which might be proven wrong, and negligence, and case after case was cited to me.

Then again every victim of a fall should be X-rayed. There *might* be a fracture even if clinically there was no sign of one. And when I had reduced a simple dislocated shoulder I was told I should have X-rayed for possible fracture of the humerus as well, although who would allow you to grip and pull on his arm if he had such a fracture?

Nor was I in sympathy with the senior surgeon's policy of 100% align-
ment in the case of fractures regardless of how long the patient had to stay
in hospital. The conversion of the patient into a resentful invalid and the
added compensation required for length of time in bed seemed not to be
considered. And when I found that a simple fracture of the fifth metacar-
pal was thought to require an open reduction *as a matter of course*, I decided there was no place in Nationalized Medicine for me and after three
months were up I left.

But before this occurred I had made the acquaintance of someone who
was going to have considerable influence on the future.* This was Lobzang
Rampa, author of *The Third Eye*, who came to visit me one afternoon at the
hospital as the result of my writing to him after reading his book. At that
time I knew nothing whatever of Tibetan Buddhism and took the story at
its face value. Only long after did I learn slowly of all the impossible events
recounted. And I liked what I saw of the author. He gave me a feeling of
confidence in some indescribable way as we talked together for an hour
in my room. In some ways this conversation helped to throw light on the
mystery of that inner compulsion that had pushed me along throughout
my life, although I told him nothing of it then. And so he left me with the
feeling that I had penetrated a little further into that dark room on the
threshold of which I had been standing before, and the darkness seemed a
little less intense.

While at the hospital I continued going to the evening meetings of the
Ouspensky groups weekly and learned much from watching them, though
it was perhaps not the sort of knowledge they imagined I was acquiring.
But if one can see oneself in other people, especially when beginning to
criticize them, then one is well on the way to feeling less contented with
oneself, for nearly always what one criticizes in another one day on another
day can be spotted in a little different form in oneself.

Once when at sea I had been talking to the Captain on the Haj who was
a very good friend and he had said, "Has anyone ever told you you are a
very selfish person, Dillon?" In fact no one had, for usually I was considered to be generous to a point of stupidity.

"No, sir, how do you mean?" I had asked.

"Because you don't allow anybody else to have any opinions of their
own. You think yours are the only right ones."

This was quite true, I had been dogmatic since early youth, but I had
never looked on this as being a selfish manifestation. Now, however, I saw

* The words "the future" replace the scratched-out words "my life."

that it was and that it was a useful tip. So now when I began to criticize someone to myself I would suddenly think how in a different way perhaps I did the same sort of thing. My Fourth Engineer friend had by now joined since he was working in London for his examination, and he showed great promise in the Work, for all the time he was deliberately trying to get to know himself in order to overcome himself. The trouble with the Gurdjieff system, as Gurdjieff himself found, is that most people are really only interested in the intellectual ideas and cosmology, not in this day to day furthering of acquaintanceship with oneself.

On Sundays when free I would go to the Mission to Seamen in Victoria Dock Road where I was well known by now since I always stayed there when in London. Not as comfortable as a good hotel, no doubt, yet all deficiencies were made up for by the warmth of the welcome to the returning seaman. The Lady Warden, the padre and his wife, the girls in the office, were all friends and sometimes I would serve in the canteen if they were short-staffed.

And now back to Oxford! How strangely the wheel of my life seemed to revolve. Instead of progressing in a straight line it seemed to rise in a spiral, each curve above smaller than the one below. Undergraduate days at Oxford came round to student days at Trinity and then came round again to Oxford for a much shorter period but in far happier circumstances. Whither was it all leading? And having Oxford again was a token that shortly there would be a new life starting elsewhere, although as yet there was no clue to it. But by now I was acutely aware of a sense of direction though the Goal was still hidden.

To be going back to Oxford in itself was a joy, and I watched eagerly from the train window for the glimpse of spires and towers ere they were blotted out by the gas-works. Then to Bradmore Road from which base of my tutor's flat I would look for digs. These I found in St. Aldate's, behind Pembroke College, right in the heart of the University as it were—and close to the Lower River, for not for long would I be able to keep away from that!

But Oxford had changed—or was it I who had changed? Perhaps a bit of both. My tutor told me that nowadays his pupils, mostly on scholarships, from grammar school, expected to be told facts that could be found in books, whereas in my day the function of the tutor was to teach how to use books and how to use one's mind, not to repeat what could be read. But they did not want to learn to think, they just wanted facts, facts and more facts. All about me in restaurants, shops and in the streets were provincial accents, mostly midland, it seemed. Did they sit up over beer till two in the morning discussing the affairs of the world as in my day, I wondered, or did they sit up with their noses in their books, just swotting? Apart from my tutor and my old schoolteacher there was no one there I knew.

Yet not feeling in the least old, on my first evening in digs I was off down to the river on the faithful blue bicycle with its white mudguards, which had seen so much of the world, and I had returned accepted as coach to one of the town clubs for whom coaches were a scarcity. They held their outings each evening and on Sundays. Before long whenever a member of the crew failed to turn up I was substituting for him in the eight, and as soon as I felt the oar again between my hands all the old reflexes returned. I could show these youngsters a thing or two about a quick recovery which is the essence of orthodox rowing, although I had now turned forty.

Next morning I started work at the DeLaWarr Laboratories, cycling about three miles through country lanes and over rustic bridges in short cuts, for they were situated outside the town on the Botley Road. There were three chief laboratories in beautifully laid out gardens and where clients were received there was a delightful little cottage with roses round the door, while the room in which Mrs. DeLaWarr worked was like an ordinary drawing room, all calculated to inspire the patient with confidence.

There I was given a little room, unfortunately with no inspiring outlook, and a "Black Box" to use with which to try and diagnose patients' diseases from the symptoms given in their letters.

The Box itself has become well known to the public since this time, through the trial at which DeLaWarr was charged with false pretenses and at which he was finally acquitted. While I was at Rizong Monastery in Ladakh in 1960 my Bristol clergyman friend sent me all the cuttings from the *Times* of the trial and I would gladly have given evidence on behalf of the Box as a Diagnostic Instrument had I been in a position to do so then, for in those next few weeks I was to test it from every angle for my own satisfaction and to find it valid for diagnosis. But naturally, as an orthodox doctor I could have nothing to do with the treatment side.

Perhaps it would be simplest if I were to record my investigations and findings which were interesting enough. Firstly, the theory of the Box is one unknown to science. By mind concentration on certain things, when they coincide with fact, an electrostatic field is set up on a rubber-covered condenser which the operator's fingers stroke and which slide over easily until such a field occurs. Then the coefficient of friction is increased and they can no longer slide but stick and the rubber crinkles up.

The ten dials are unnecessary. Theoretically they are for setting against different numbers representing different parts of the body diseases, causes, etc., and they do make a little difference to the friction when it is produced, but not enough to merit the trouble in setting them each time. The Box can be worked without them by anyone with sufficient sensitivity, but they do add to the selling power.

Mrs. DeLaWarr had a keen sensitivity and worked the Box easily and I began by running through a few cases she had already done and comparing my results with hers and found them approximating. Then I started work on my own cases, reading the accompanying letter complaining of certain signs and symptoms, seeing the name of the writer and then concentrating on the name together with the items on the cards one worked through, starting with the anatomy card, then the detailed anatomy of any part which had caused friction and on to diseases, bacteria, etc. until one had an entire case examination made out.

But it was not long before I began to wonder whether my knowing as a doctor what might be wrong from reading of the complaints did not influence the friction of "stick," as it is called. It could do so by my unconsciously exerting a shade greater pressure on the rubber. This must be investigated, so one morning I took a letter and looked at the name and address and no more, putting it back carefully in its envelope so that I should not see anything suggestive. Then I began to work in the usual way and found the nasal organ was the part affected but by no allergy; a bacterium seemed to be the cause and the bacterium itself came up strongly. This made no sense, unless the patient merely suffered from a common cold. I decided not to waste more time but to look at the letter and find out what the woman really was complaining of.

"Dear Mrs. DeLaWarr, I have been suffering from nasal catarrh for a long time now and although I have had all sorts of anti-allergic drugs and injections nothing seems to do it any good . . ."

To say I was amazed would be to put it mildly. Next day I tried again with a letter from a Colonel and osteo-arthritis came up and in the letter he complained of arthritis. There was no need to assume any more that it was my imagination that was producing the "stick."

The spot of blood on blotting paper I never used, for it was quite unnecessary if one concentrated on the name of the patient, which was preferable to concentrating on the blood.

But one of the scientific objections to the Box was that a small percentage of persons were unable to use it, through lack of sensitivity. The "too materialistic" as DeLaWarr called them, [and he] himself never seemed to use it. It occurred to me one day, therefore, that if there was anything in the dial numbers there should be a "Booster Rate" which would emphasize all "sticks" so I set about trying to find this, turning the first dial and thinking "booster" until a "stick" came and then leaving it turned on and going on to the next dial and so on until a five figure number had come up and no more were significant.

Having run through an anatomy card of a patient in the usual way and produced certain results, I then put up the Booster Rate and went through it again. Sure enough, the coefficient of friction was much increased in all those items which had produced some before and a few extra items also showed. It seemed that there might be something in it. So without telling her why I asked Mrs. DeLaWarr to run through the same anatomy card for the same patient and, after I had jotted down her results which were similar to mine, I put up the Booster Rate and asked her to do it again. At once she exclaimed at the greater friction and found even more extra items than I had (these extra items could be disregarded for clinical purposes as being too subliminal). Then I explained what I had done, and it but remained to try it out on someone who was unable to work the instrument normally.

Periodically science or medical students would come out from the University to see the place and these were always allowed to test the Box. A fortnight or so later a group arrived and all but three were able to get some results from it, but these three could not make any friction. When, however, the Booster Rate was set without their having been told why, they achieved the same results as the rest. It did work! Hence if the Booster Rate were incorporated in the Box of the future it would make the rest of the dials unnecessary and would ensure that anyone could work it. The theory of it may have been based on a hypothesis unprovable by science but, at least within the hypothesis, it followed quite logically and coherently.

The corollary of this discovery was naturally that the Rate should also Boost the healing instruments but there I could and would do nothing. Diagnosis was one thing and treatment was another. During our medical course we had been told, "Diagnosis is a hit-or-miss affair. You can never be certain of your diagnosis until the case comes to post mortem," so that any improvement on this should be welcome even if not as yet scientifically demonstrable. Moreover sometimes it is impossible to make any diagnosis. In such a case the Box is invaluable. Naturally measles, typhoid, a bone fracture and the like do not need it. But in many types of illness there are causes which are not manifest, especially in the psychological field and medical science is beginning to realize some of the diseases which are primarily caused by psychological responses, such as coronary, pentic ulcer, dermatitis, blood pressure, and many others. The Box can determine such psychological causes much more easily than can the psychiatrist and with less ill effects on the patient.

A point that was made at the trial but which met with little sympathetic response was that the Box could predict the onset of a disease a few years before its clinical manifestation. And this was the reason; apparently Mr. DeLaWarr would not have the Box tested although this could still have been done successfully on some case already known clinically.

This was not a thing that could itself be put to the test since a disease might be two or three years or more before showing even if the Box did diagnose it. In fact it is well known that tuberculosis shows no clinical symptoms for at least a year after it has begun, which is why x-rays of chests and spines may be negative and yet in time tuberculosis will show there. It was not until after the trial was over that I myself had astonishing evidence of the truth of this claim, however.

One day in the laboratory when I had no official work to do I amused myself running through some of my friends and seeing what, if anything, might be wrong with them. One of these was my Oxford tutor. Up came the heart very strongly on the anatomy sheet, and on turning to diseases, coronary thrombosis was elicited, left-side (for the Box will give the greatest detail). So strong was the friction that I felt alarmed and then decided to put the Box away for the day and try it again on the morrow. Once again came up the same trouble just as strongly. I went out and rung up Mrs. McKie as casually as possible on some pretext and then asked after Jimmy's health. He was perfectly well. I told her what I had done and suggested she should keep an eye on his heart in case the Box was right, but I said nothing about the enormous friction as I did not want to alarm her. When she asked for copies of my two diagnoses of her self and him I watered his down considerably. That was in 1957.

Some time in 1959 he had his first coronary and in 1960, on the day I left my Ladakhi monastery, he died of a second thrombosis. Pure coincidence? It could be certainly. More cases need testing and the results keeping for a few years to see. But it is significant.

May Morning came and I met Mrs. McKie on Magdalene Bridge to listen once more—and for the last time it seems, to the choir welcoming in the Spring. In the evening, to celebrate my birthday I gave a dinner and a theater to the McKies and to my old schoolmistress. They had never met before although both had heard often of the other, and unfortunately circumstances compelled the friendship that sprung up to be a temporary affair.

Every evening would see me down on the river either coaching from the bank or the boat. When Eights week came in June I was able to watch the Bumping Races for the first time since I had been an undergraduate, and later again to attend the Town Regatta and also to escort my crew to Stratford-on-Avon for a regatta there.

Oxford in spring and early summer cannot be bettered. The cherry blossom is coming out along Parks Road, and the North Oxford Gardens are among some of the finest in England and please the eye of the passerby. The grass at Marston is long and emerald green besprinkled with tall buttercups and little fleecy clouds saunter slowly over the sky as you lie on your back in a punt and gaze up at them, puffing at your pipe, and the world seems to be quite a good place after all.

But the next day is Monday and you are back at work again. Naturally incurables numbered greatly among the clients for, if orthodox medicine would not cure them, they had the right to seek where they could to hold on to life, and we had quite a high percentage of disseminated sclerosis cases. To my surprise, when testing these, in every case the same cause was elicited, the *haemoplilus influenzae* bacillus situated in the subarachnoid space of the brain, and, in advanced cases, also present in the third ventricles. And when I told Mrs. DeLaWarr she said she always found the same.

Now this would be easily verifiable by post mortem on a case which had died of disseminated sclerosis, in the interests of finding a cure for future sufferers. Again, too, swayback in sheep is allied to this disease, scientifically proven, so that it is possible that a sick sheep's post mortem may show the subarachnoid space there affected too. At all events, if it is ever so discovered, the Box will have to be taken much more seriously by science than hitherto.

Another interesting piece of evidence given by the Box was the difference in origins between rheumatoid and osteo-arthritis. The former appeared to be due to a bacillus affecting the red bone marrow primarily and the latter an allergic reaction affecting the white bone marrow abetted always by some psychological upset. Certainly this Box would merit further investigation to see if it really can aid some of the problems medical science cannot as yet solve.

For the much vaunted camera, on the other hand, I had no time. It could be made to work only by one person, the lab man in charge of it, and this had been proved many, many times. Moreover, as was brought out in the trial, the photographs resulting much more resembled a layman's woolly conception of anatomy than the real thing, and the lab man had no knowledge of anatomy.

How then did he do it? In DeLaWarr's library was a book published in 1913 by some Japanese scientists, recording the results of investigation into thought photography. They had found that a medium, holding a plate and concentrating on something, could produce that thing's picture on the plate quite clearly. This may seem strange since science has not thought to research on the possibilities of thought photography even as it has no conception of the scope of the mind's action as is known to, and taken for granted by, the East. At all events this lab man is admittedly psychic and also frightened of his own abilities in that direction, but it was to his interest to keep the working of the camera in his own hands. This point was also made at the trial.

At first I was happy there and interested in this unorthodox sort of research. I was also able to check clinically many patients against the findings of the Box, and tried to make my investigation as nearly orthodox as possible. For there was so much here that deserved careful examination of the fundamentals, going slowly step by step, that there was no need whatever for reaching for the moon in the shape of even more spectacular results with which to "make history." It is possible that the fact that nothing was an original invention of DeLaWarr's that caused such ambition, yet modifications and exploration would have been far more valuable, provided that each step was checked and rechecked and a single instance was not regarded as being sufficient cause for bursting into print.

It was due to DeLaWarr being carried away by his vain enthusiasm and ambition that ultimately led to my departure from the Laboratories. When I had started there I had been warned that my terms of service might end abruptly at any time since the financial situation was precarious, despite appearances being to the contrary. Hence this was made the excuse for giving me notice a week or so after I had refused point blank to write up the results of an experiment that had hardly yet been made, unwisely adding a few pungent remarks on scientific honesty versus spectacular claims.

Mrs. DeLaWarr had no part or parcel in any of this. She was a woman of great compassion and genuinely desired to help sufferers and was quite contented to work the Box and treatment instruments and she may well have been successful in a number of cases simply by the force of her personality. That there was a great deal of work there to be done, seemed certain, since our medicine, "modern" though we think it, is really primitive in the extreme, since we have lost all knowledge of the connection between mind and body and do not know except in the most glaring cases, such as duodenal ulcer, how they interact.

Later I was to learn something of the physiological effects produced by deep meditation, which would be quite inexplicable by ordinary means. Indeed, their very existence is unknown to Western medical men, but the power of the mind over the so-called autonomic nervous system, as well as over the sympathetic, can be demonstrated by Yogis who have made it a lifetime practice.

While a little sorry to be leaving Oxford, yet it seemed as if this interlude, also, had served its turn. I had had the enjoyment of Oxford again quite unexpectedly and wondered what the next turn of the spiral would bring.

My suitcase packed, I looked out on Tom Tower (which could only be seen from the lavatory window) and Pembroke College and St. Aldate's Church for the last time. I had been going to St. Aldate's on Sunday mornings to see if my memory of those undergraduate-stirring services was accurate. But hands had changed and it now seemed to be catering more for the town and far less for the gown and lacked the vigor of former days.

By this time much of my interest in orthodox religion had gone. The idea of a Savior who died for men and not a Teacher who died as the result of man's stupidity and cruelty, irked. I had ceased to believe what the Church taught although what Christ Himself had taught, as expressed in the Gospels, seemed of the highest order. Christ had said: "Not all who say unto Me, 'Lord, Lord!' shall enter into the Kingdom of Heaven." Yet I had been told from childhood that all the aunts and all their friends would go to Heaven because they went to church every Sunday and said their prayers twice daily. And certainly they all believed it. But so many of the parables seemed to suggest that man had to do a great deal for himself before he would be passed as acceptable to God. The foolish Virgins, the Ten Talents, the Sheep and the Goats, the Pearl of Great Price, and so on, in none of these was the central figure a passive agent. Christ seemed to have come to give a message to man, a system whereby he might evolve a little spiritually and it had been distorted into the doctrine that belief in Him would cleanse us from all sins and bring us to Heaven. Later I was to come to the view that Christ was a Bodhisattva of a very high order who gained Buddhahood on the cross when He said sincerely, "Father, forgive them, they know not what they do," for that is said to be the peak of Bodhisattvaship, when a man can die slowly under torture and feel no hatred for his torturers the while. But at that time I had never heard the word "Bodhisattva" and did not know the concept other than as that of Teacher and Master-Teacher, which is in effect what the Bodhisattva is.*

Since it was now July another cycle trip seemed called for, before old age crept on. G. was contacted and we met in Folkestone and stayed the night at what had been the aunts' boarding house, sharing a great brass knobbed double bed, and next day we were on the cross channel steamer for France.

This time I had made to myself a "Work-aim" that nothing that happened on the trip would upset me. This would be considered by members of the Group as far too big an aim, and one impossible of keeping, in fact a foolish project. But because I had given myself time to become accustomed to the idea before starting, I began the journey almost looking forward to some trouble as a challenge. And, sure enough, it started right away; for we slept past our station for changing and were carried on to Germany instead of Basel and when we discovered it we had to buy a ticket back to the point of change.

"I thought you would be furious and letting off steam," said G. in the cold light of dawn, as we shivered on a seat on an open platform. So I told him about the Work and Work-Aims. He was interested but only with his Reason; it did not appeal to his Emotions, so that he did not take it up; but he admitted there must be something in it to have made such a difference in one like myself who had always blown off steam at low pressure and then forgotten about it immediately after, and failed to understand why the other person did not forget too! G. of course never minded, but others who did not know me, did. And this insensitivity was something to be observed and overcome.

We reached Milan and then left the station in pouring rain. Indeed the whole trip was marred by periodic thunderstorms, but all the same it was enjoyable. The terrain was flat for we were covering the Lombardy Plain, going to Ravenna, first and then up to Venice and back through Padua, Verona and Bologna, all names of fame in the world of letters and thought of the past. At Padua the old university gates were locked at the early hour we arrived but we climbed up them and looked over to imagine Erasmus walking in the shade of the trees in the gardens.

It is pleasant after a hard day's cycling to eat one's supper in the cool evening air (forgetting about the mosquitoes) and to light one's pipe before stretching out a weary body on a soft bed of cut grass, there to watch the

---

* The phrase "which is in effect what the Bodhisattva is" is added to the sentence by hand.

stars, as first Venus shines forth and then one tiny star appears. Suddenly there is a cluster around it, which was not there a moment before, and now another twinkles and another, until the sky is dark and full of lights. Some of the constellations I had learned from my Captain on the Haj and these I would identify to G. as he lay beside me more than half asleep from a strenuous day so different from his office work. Or we would go over the day's adventures of which there is no room here to tell and I talked to him, too, of Lobzang Rampa who had had so strange an effect on me.

For there was something to look forward to on our return: Rampa had written to suggest my coming over for a week or two's holiday, since he had a flat in Howth overlooking Dublin Bay and Ireland's Eye. Whatever was said of him in the future I felt that he was the man who held the key to my next move.

Thus it came about I was leaning on the ship's rail as she tied up at Dublin Wall, but the roadway was invisible from there. All night I had been turning over in my mind my past meeting with Rampa. Had I built too much on it? Was my feeling of trust in him misplaced? Whether he was really a Tibetan Lama or not did not trouble me, I accepted things as they purported to be, for he was not the sort of man you met every day. Had I known as much about Tibetan Buddhism then as I know now, and about the lives of Lamas, I might have missed much by rejecting the contact, on the grounds of spurious claims, and that loss would have been immeasurable as it turned out.

Down the gangway I went and through the sheds into the road. There he was, standing on the opposite curb, a strange, lonely figure, and I felt at once that my confidence had not been misplaced.

For the next two weeks we were much together. We went out in a hired dinghy with outboard engine and explored the cliffs and islands; we ran round the countryside in a car and all the time we talked. Much of what he told me purporting to be of his life I now know to be false, because life in Tibetan monasteries is not like that, but what he said of the Universe and man's place in it made good sense and merely continued my own line of thinking. And some of what he told me of myself was to be repeated in various forms by three other persons in three different countries, one of them a clairvoyant Hindu in India.

Moreover he had quite definitely psychic powers well developed in certain directions and during this time he aided the development of my own, although heretofore I had imagined I was not in the least psychic nor had I ever had any desire to be. Although I did not stay in the flat because there was not room, but in a hotel at the end of the road, he was able to influence my dreams and I had experiences of a kind that can be read of under the heading of "astral traveling" of which at that time I knew nothing.

The day before I was due to leave to return and look for another ship, he took me for a long car drive in the evening.

"Do one more sea voyage and then go to India and look for a monastery where you can learn meditation, Michael," he said.

A monastery! I had never thought of a monastic life before, knowing it only from the Christian Orders that one had seen at Oxford. And a Christian monastery would be no good since one would have to be orthodox and a believer in Mother Church. A Tibetan monastery then? In India? Yes, there were some, he said. Meditation was the key to my future. I should practice it. The idea of a monastery, too, appealed.*

With new thoughts and new experiences, I returned to tramp Leadenhall and Fenchurch Street, looking for a job for with all my commitments I had to continue to earn. Young G.'s school reports were excellent and justified the change made, since he was good at games as well as work, and his Latin was especially good. The kitty was being put to continual use and that young Irish hospital patient was happy in a new job. All was well with the world!

Ellerman's had only the *City of Bath*, still on the same run and requiring a new crew but not before the end of November. I was not interested. But in vain I went to office after office, even of companies with white crews, but could find no vacancy. Then Ellerman informed me they wanted a relieving surgeon for the *City of Port Elizabeth*, one of their big South African ships, but only for coasting on the continent to unload and load. It would be a three weeks job and I took it rather than hang around any longer with nothing.

Naturally the crew was greatly reduced for many had gone on leave and only the bare essential number were left, including but a single apprentice. Forthwith I told the Mate I had had experience of mooring and casting off on the *Bath* and would he like an assistant on the fo'c'sle? He would! This ship had a telephone communication with the bridge, more modern than the old *Bath* with her megaphone, and I must relay his remarks through that. He was English, fortunately and by now I would be less likely to mistake what he said.

The Master of the ship was the Commodore of the fleet and the day after we had sailed at lunch he told me that the Pilot had said to him, "I thought you said there would be only one officer on the bridge but you

* The last sentence, "the idea of a monastery, too, appealed," is added by hand.

seem to have two and they're both three-stripers." And to that he had replied with a grin:

"Yes, it's all right, that's our apprentice surgeon!"

He was amused at my enthusiasm which kept me up sometimes half the night and at others got me out of my bunk in the small hours of the morning, but he seemed to approve.

It was when we were in Antwerp having a quiet night that towards morning I had a very vivid dream of that old schoolmistress friend in Oxford, now quite an elderly lady. She appeared in deep distress and wanted to talk to me but there were too many people around so I suggested we went back to her house. On the day I awoke, but so vivid remained her distress that at once I wrote and asked her if anything was wrong, telling her of this dream, and its date.

She wrote back by return and said that on the evening before she had been thinking about me and had wanted to talk to me badly, but I had gone off she did not know where and she had been quite upset about it. As she had never been a good correspondent, we seldom wrote more than about twice a year so there had been no reason for me letting her know I was on a short trip. But this telepathy, although received about twelve hours *post eventum*, was the direct effect of the work Rampa, now "Grampa Rampa," had put in. Would that it had continued but in fact psychic powers should not be sought for their own sake, as is the teaching of the Tibetan Lamas themselves. If they come they come, usually through meditation, and they should be ignored and only used to help others' progress. If they are pursued then they become a cul-de-sac and inhibit any further spiritual development, which is the main aim.

Back in London there were still no vacancies and finally I reluctantly accepted the *City of Bath* for another contract period, knowing that my old Captain would be one of those being relieved, unfortunately. As things turned out it would have been a great boon had he and Willie been on her when the reporters arrived!

CHAPTER 12

The Last Voyage

I had one more week with Grampa Rampa before leaving for New York on the French ship *Liberté*, with the relieving crew. In that week he talked still more and put many new ideas into my head that proved worthy of the space allotted them. On the last night he saw me off from Dun Laoghaire Pier for Holyhead, and I felt much moved at the thought of the parting. One last handshake and I turned abruptly and did not look back.

In New York we had five days to wait, for the *Bath* had gone South to Norfolk, Newport News, Boston, Baltimore and Philadelphia to load for India as was her usual itinerary, and now she was lying in the latter port. My bicycle had come with me, inevitably, and now, on a Sunday, I astonished New York by cycling all around the town, not aware till after that bicycles, anywhere but in the great Park, are quite unknown in that city. Luckily it was Sunday or traffic would have been very heavy and there are lights at the corners of every block.

Two other noteworthy visits were paid, one to UN headquarters, that curious piece of architecture, which stands up like a child's block left lying on the floor, and you expect that any moment something will knock it down. We saw the various committee rooms, shown by a most attractive guide who refused to be led into controversial subjects such as Suez, started by an American and defended by myself.

The second place visited was the Planetarium and well deserving of a visit it is. Being early December there were lectures going on under the revolving Heaven, but unfortunately the lecturer going unscientifically insisted on dwelling on the hypothetical Star of Bethlehem as the main theme of his lecture. But the *piece de resistance* was the largest meteorite in the world that was discovered in Siberia in 1908. It came from outer space, no one knows whence. As I stood and gazed at it an odd feeling developed in me—pure fancy you may say if you like—that in its natural habitat it had been regarded as being alive and it was at a loss to understand why here, on Earth, it was thought to be but an inert lump of metal. Children were climbing over it and I had the feeling that it was appealing for some understanding that it was as alive as they.

This may sound fanciful in the extreme but wait a moment! Time and space are purely relative to man's SIZE. A spider runs across the floor at 100 miles an hour covering about ten miles while we cross the same distance of about four yards in the same time in four or five steps. An ant cannot comprehend a man, only the hills and dales and forests of the shoe it walks on. If man was transferred to a planet where time was much faster than it is here, he would appear an inert, lifeless thing and his movements would not be perceptible. If to a planet where time was much slower than on Earth, then all things that to us appear inert, would be seen to be in motion.

When I was a medical student I once read an American book, which was a *Symposium of Science* for the current year (possibly 1949). It was a thin green book and I only remember one single sentence out of it: "In a hydrogen atom the relative distance of the electron from its nucleus is *twice the relative distance* of the earth from the sun."

This had at once struck a chord. Space was relative to our size. The atom is beyond our vision being too small yet it has greater space in it than our own solar system—and hydrogen the smallest of the atoms.

The converse naturally followed in my mind: Suppose the earth was but an electron on the atom of some entity so great that it does not exist for us any more than we exist for the ant, nay, rather for the virus? This idea I put forth periodically and found it made very little impression; yet to me it seemed a stupendous thought. Hence I maintain that my feeling that the meteorite was really alive and merely appeared to us to be inert, is not so fantastic after all. Has any one with the power of psychometry laid a hand on it to see what information can be ascertained? If it is beyond the bounds of science to find out its history one might as well use these methods themselves that go beyond science to explain.

The *City of Bath* arrived and I was back again in the same cabin I had left some years before at crack of dawn when accompanied to the nursing home in Calcutta by the Second Mate. When unpacked I went up the stairs to see my old Captain. He was standing with his back to the door and instead of knocking I said, "Hallo, sir!"

He looked round in surprise, "Hal-lo, Dillon, you back again? Come on in and sit down, what'll you have to drink? I am afraid I have no Irish or rum. Will it be gin or sherry? No use offering you Scotch." By which he indicated he remembered all about me and was pleased to see me again!

"I'll never forget the day I saw you up the Sampson post," he said as we raised glasses.

"Maybe I'll be up it again, sir," I replied, fully intending to get down to work as soon as possible and hoping there would be a cooperative Mate. The Sampson posts held the lights over the after hatches for cargo-working at night and the glass covers had been in need of cleaning. In height they were level with the Bridge and he had been tickled to see me up there one day polishing the glass.

The Mate turned out to be a very nice chap but unfortunately he was leaving and a new one was being flown out. He said he had cramps in his legs and wanted treatment, but in fact he admitted later he anticipated trouble on the ship and did not want to sail with her.

Further, the carpenter it seemed had gone ashore one evening and been knocked down by a taxi in New York and was in hospital with a broken leg so a new Chips was also being flown out. Meanwhile he welcomed a spare hand to assist the two apprentices.

When the new Mate came aboard the old one brought him to the hatch and he peered down to see myself and one apprentice screwing down the covers of the water tanks held by innumerable nuts all round. When the new Chips arrived I was battening down the after hatches at the top of the gangway so that he came straight up to me and demanded to know if I was the carpenter. When I denied it without telling him who I was he walked away in perplexity, made even worse by a kalassie claiming I was the surgeon.

But the happy state of the ship did not last. The new captain had a reputation amongst the officers and it was this that had led the Mate from experience to secede. As far as we had seen him on the *Liberté*, he had been a charming, paternal type of man, with two more years only to go before retirement. But it was to happen that whenever we met a company's ship in a port inevitably we were asked "Who's your Old Man?" and when we said [who it was] there were whistles and questions as to whether there was trouble on board. For a long time all was well in that respect and I could see no reason for this, and defended him.

On the other hand the new Mate's character can be judged from almost his first action on board, which was to send for the two apprentices in his cabin and when they came, standing nervously at the door, for he was their lord and master, he looked them up and down and then said:

"I had a bloody hell of a time when I was apprentice and I'm going to make damned sure you do too. Now go!"

Finally the Purser was out to save and when the passengers left we were fed worse than on any other of the company's ships I had been in, so that complaints and abuse became rife. But as yet all this was in the future.

This was the layout for the voyage in which the *Sunday Express* was suddenly to tell the world about my past history.

We took on seven passengers in New York and sailed for St. John's where we were to spend Christmas. The Seamen's Club, not being part of the Mission to Seamen, closed itself on Christmas Day so that its workers could have Christmas at home. At Victoria Dock Road in London, there would be great festivities making it as much as possible a home from home event for all seamen in port. There would be a present for every comer, a proper dinner, games and dancing, evening chapel for those who wished and finally country dancing. As it was, with all on shore closed, we drank on board most of the day, or the others did, while I read a Billy Bunter book which my doctor friend sent yearly, knowing my infantile taste and loyalty to Frank Richards of *Gem* and *Magnet* fame. There was of course a big dinner of about nine courses provided by the company and it was snowing outside to aid the Christmas spirit which was not, however, very much in evidence.

At length we sailed for India with eight passengers. One of them described himself as a Food Expert, and even had his notepaper headed thus. His sole topic of conversation was food and drink and he said he had a library of over a thousand books all on food. When we reached Bombay he returned to the ship shortly in disgust saying that he could not get a decent whiskey ashore because of the permit system—as if he had come to India to drink whiskey which he could have got more easily at home!

In Bombay I went ashore on my bicycle mindful of the search for a meditation center and without the faintest idea how to set about finding such a thing. At the time I had never heard of Burmese centers or Theravadin Buddhism and the only Buddhism I had met at all was in *The Wisdom of India* by Lin Yu Tung, which I had picked up in a single volume with the *Wisdom of China* in New York. Herein the extract from the *Suranagama Sutra* had struck me as surpassing anything the West had yet produced on the problem of Perception; it was pure metaphysics but as yet Buddhism as such was still a closed book; nor was I interested in it, not even in its Tibetan version, although I had read one or two travel books on Tibet recently, stimulated by *The Third Eye*.

Wandering round a bookshop I happened on a guide to India which looked possibly useful and therein was to find largely advertised a place called Bodh Gaya of which I had never heard. Apparently, from the pictures, it had a big temple of an architectural type which I had not seen before and it might be interesting. If I could get a weekend off in Calcutta, it was only an overnight's train's journey.

Meanwhile deck work had flagged and slowly petered out. The Mate was hostile and although at first he gave me a few small chipping jobs he became more and more inimical. The apprentices suffered most. Their cabin, mine and the Pursers' were below decks in an alley together so naturally I tended to throw in my lot with them who were next door, since the Purser also was unfriendly, so that unless I went topside to join the deck officers over drinks I tended to share the off time of the apprentices.

Things came to a head one day when the Mate, having seen us playing deck tennis after tea one Sunday quite legitimately, called the senior apprentice and gave a list of bans, including that neither of them should play deck tennis at all and that they should not be seen around with me. This was the last straw and the apprentice went to the Old Man and asked him whether he upheld the ruling. At this time the captain had showed no signs of living up to his reputation and was kindly and jovial, with passengers to keep him amused.

Now he asked the apprentice quietly, "How long has this been going on?"

"Ever since the Mate came on board, sir," said the boy and then told him how they had been greeted. After that things improved a little and we could go on playing but the Mate, who had had orders to stop his persecution, was burning inside with even greater hatred. He had suffered from a bad Mate himself in his apprentice days when apprentices could be beaten for their peccadilloes, and instead of learning therefore to lessen the sufferings of others he had built up inside him a resentment which could only be assuaged by seeing others suffer, and being no longer allowed to beat he thought up all other varieties of irritations and annoyances.

It was on this voyage, having nothing to do, that I wrote the *Rishi Stories* in much the same manner as the *Poems* had been written and adding drawings at the beginning and end of each section.

In Calcutta permission was readily given for me to go away for a weekend and I took a first class ticket to Gaya, nearest station to this famous place called Bodh Gaya. It was the first and last time I traveled first class, for later as a monk I was not to be able to afford more than a third class ticket. At sea most officers wore lungis for night wear, that check cotton strop of cloth of the Moslem wrapped around like a skirt, since most of the Indian crew had them too, and they were very comfortable. Unaware at that time that everyone in India travels with his bedding, I had taken only a handbag with my towel and lungi for the night. In the carriage with me were three very Westernized Indians who laid out their bedrolls with linen sheets and donned their silken pyjamas. I put on my lungi and stripped to the waist as it was hot, and stretched out on the seat with my bag under my head as pillow. Here was a reversal of the usual sahib status!

At Gaya it was possible to rent a bed in a rest room in the station, a notable invention of Indian Railways, and when once cleaned, fed and rested I set out by cycle rickshaw for Bodh Gaya miles away, the rickshaw wallah charging the poor sucker with blue eyes four rupees instead of the statuary fare of one! But the rickshaw wallahs in India are exploited and 1/6 for a seven mile cycle pulling a carriage behind you is hardly adequate, especially since, if the locals take it, they may pile the rickshaw full of luggage and children as well and the 1/6 is supposed to cover the hire of the vehicle however many are in it.

It was late afternoon as I rattled, rather than bowled, along. We had negotiated the town on whose streets are gathered the greatest motley of pedestrian traffic that can perhaps be seen anywhere. Cows with their calves, goats with their kids, dogs with their puppies, hens with their chickens, and women looking after their children, all in a mêlée in the middle of the road, wandering about without regard to anything except their private business, mostly, the eternal search for fodder.

Outside the town it became more peaceful and plains flanked the road and a river could be seen in the distance. By the wayside sat a beggarwoman extending the stumps of her arms, her hands having been cut off. Had she lost them in an accident or had she been punished by a jealous husband or what was her story? I wondered. Always she sat there and I was to see her in future years when visiting the place again.

Further on still was an elephant at work, decorated with a great bead necklace and hauling treetops, stacked on its back. That also was a permanent feature of this road.

I wondered what lay ahead knowing that something did and I kept an eye on the horizon for sight of that great Temple depicted in the guidebook. At least it appeared for a moment and then was hidden again by trees; we had reached the village of Bodh Gaya and here the rickshaw journey ended, I should have to walk the rest.

Up a hill through what might have justifiably been called the "High Street" one comes out suddenly on a broad plateau and there, to the left, on sunken ground reached by steps stands the Buddhist Temple. A wireless blaring an advertisement for a Gaya cinema struck a jarring note and I hurried down the steps to escape from it.

At the bottom as I stood looking at the Temple I had my first sight of a Tibetan "Lama," just like the pictures in those travel books I had recently been reading. He was old and wrinkled, clad in a long dirty red robe over an equally dirty skirt. He had cloth boots also of red but brighter, and an oddly shaped hat or cap on his head. As he passed, he looked at me and I stared back, unable to believe I was looking at a real Tibetan.

Before I had finished examining the architecture he had come round again for he seemed to be walking round the Temple, and again we stared at each other. I missed the opportunity. But if he came round a third time I would try and stop him and talk. He did. I approached with a smile and at once his dirty face wrinkled up into a friendly grin. I held out my hand, quite unaware that more than half the world does not have the practice of shaking hands. He looked at it a moment then swinging his arm out he swept his hand into mine with a mighty clap.

"Are you a Tibetan Lama?" I asked.

His grin increased. "Tibet," he said.

There the conversation perforce ended for it seemed he did not speak English, and after an awkward moment [of] my not knowing what to do or say, he raised both hands, palms together, to his chin and gave a little bow and resumed his walk.

After examining all that was to be seen and noting that there was a strange oriental looking building which had a notice to say it was a Tibetan Temple I decided to go back to my room for the night and return first thing in the morning for it was dusk and I did not fancy a rickshaw in the dark.

At the top of the hill I saw a sight that sickened me. A concourse of men were coming up led by one who was dragging a dog along by its hind legs, face down in the dust. I felt that it was alive though it gave no sign and was on the verge of jumping forward and intervening when I remembered how I had once tried to intervene with the maltreatment of a horse in France when on a cycle trip and had been defeated by the language and had only been able to swear at them in English and cause much laughter. Out here they would not take kindly to a foreigner intervening anyway. At that moment as I was uncertain what to do a "Lama" came out from a shop and gave a start towards the dog, but seeing me he stopped and gazed curiously at my blue eyes. I hurried on hoping that he would manage to reassure the beast, since he might know the language and the people. The Hindus who pride themselves so on not killing animals for food are utterly callous with regard to their sufferings and I have seen more cruelty to animals in India than anywhere else in the world—but then I have not visited Spain which I have heard is also pretty bad.

Next morning I woke with a feeling of suppressed excitement. Something was going to happen today which would have some bearing on my future, of that I was sure and after breakfast in the station restaurant I was out to be pounced on by the rickshaw wallah of the night before who must have been up at dawn to be ready to make such easy money. He had incipient elephantiasis of the left leg, a very common sight in India, so that when the true fare was revealed I did not feel too badly about the unnecessary expenditure.

The excitement built up inside me as we covered the seven miles again. Today I would meet someone who would help me to the next step. Who would it be? And there was the Tibetan temple to be seen, the first of its kind encountered outside books.

On the plateau I went to a house with a notice over it saying Maha Bodhi Society, Bookshop. The name meant nothing then though it was to become so familiar. But the man behind the counter, in the long shirt and *dhoti* of the Indian, spoke English well.

After a look at the books I told him I was searching for a monastery where I could stay for some time and learn meditation. At this he went outside and peered around. Then he signed to me to stay where I was and went over to a tea stall across the road and returned with what must surely be a Tibetan. But . . .

"Good Lord, the fellow's dressed like a woman!" was my astonished thought. He was a short, thin man with yellow skin and heavily hooded eyes and shaven head. He wore a yellow sleeveless shirt with stand-up

Chinese type collar and a yellow scarf tucked in it. Below was a dark chocolate skirt, slit a little way up at the sides to show a crimson silk lining.
Western socks and shoes completed the outfit. Later I was to know that
this was his "undress uniform," being merely out for a cup of tea he had
not put on his outer robe or top skirt, without which, strictly speaking, one
should not appear in public, but which is very commonly done in the heat
of India, near one's residence.

"This is the Abbot of the Tibetan Monastery," said the Indian book-
seller, stressing the word "Abbot" to show that he was a man to be greatly
respected.

I held out my hand shyly, still not knowing that it was just "not done."
But the Tibetans in India have learned this curious habit of shaking hands
done by foreigners and Westernized Indians and he readily shook it, and
spoke in Hindi. But the Malim's Sahib's Hindustani, useful for ships, was
far removed from social conversation ashore and I could not understand.
So he flapped his hand up and down twice and then dashed off at a run,
calling to two youths walking across the grass. The elder turned out to be
an interpreter and together we went into the Tibetan monastery and up to
the "Abbot" or Head Lama's room.

He was Dhardoh Rimpoche (pronounced Dun-do) who spent three
months of the year here and the rest running a school for Tibetan children
in Kalimpong, it seemed. Tea and biscuits were served and then he invited
me to stay the night at the Maha Bodhi rest house next door, as his guest
and to have supper with him. So promising to return shortly I went back
to the station to relinquish the rest room there and fetch my bag and spent
the afternoon in the Tibetan Monastery with the monks who were sitting
cross-legged on the floor of a room all engaged in needlework, making
and stitching colored fringes on to beautiful brocade cloth for purposes
unknown. They tried to talk to me in Hindi and we managed a little. Then
the inevitable Tibetan tea was served, and this was my first taste of that
commodity, salted and buttered. It had a smoky flavor, and was not too
salty and the butter not rancid as books on Tibet always make a point of its
being and I liked it. The odd thing was that I felt perfectly at home here, a
feeling quite inexplicable.

Later Dhardoh Rimpoche showed me all around Bodh Gaya as well
as his own monastery and then we went back to supper in his room. This
consisted of a strange kind of soup with lumps of dough in it and a dish of
what looked like leather, but turned out to be the famous dried yak meat,
which I found quite impossible to eat, so tough was it. He also showed me
how to mix tsampa flour in the tea and mold it with the fingers and then

eat the sodden mess. But it seemed almost impossible to get rid of since it clung to my upper palate and finally I had to surreptitiously put a finger in to scoop it down or my mouth would not hold any more. I never did get used to this article of diet. Finally he gave me a card and told me to come to him in Kalimpong when I would be free.

A lay Tibetan took me across to the Maha Bodhi Rest house and, anxious to find a urinal I asked him where the lavatory was. The youth looked at me in astonishment and waved his hand to signify that one could do what one would anywhere. But it seemed rather sacrilegious to commit a nuisance in a monastery garden so I set about investigating on my own and eventually found what I sought.

Next morning trumpets awoke me early, odd sounding trumpets, nothing like the reveille of bugles, and looking out of the window I saw everywhere Tibetan monks all in their best robes, it seemed, and tall yellow hats with fringes on, curved like a horn. Those were worn by those who were blowing trumpets and conch shells. Hastily putting on shirt and trousers and my blazer because it was cold outside, being only the first of March, I went out to see what this was all about. Then Dhardoh Rimpoche emerged with a dark red outer robe and red skirt and a camera swinging from his hand. He signed to me to join him.

The monks now assembled in a double line and then three brought a glass case with a Buddha image in it raised on a kind of chair, carried aloft and this seemed to be the central figure of the procession. The Head Lama himself did not join the procession that then set off to circumambulate the great temple but stayed with me making ready his camera to photograph it as it came round the other side, as I did too, for this would be a picture of pictures! I would send a copy to Grampa Rampa!

The procession over there followed, per impossible, a sort of sports day program. The monks stripped to the waist and appeared in little shorts, the usual striped underwear in India, and disappeared down the road, while Rimpoche and myself climbed upon the roof of the monastery to watch the foot race. It must have been about half a mile long and soon they were pounding down the road and in the monastery garden until the winner arrived at Dhardoh Rimpoche's place, followed by the rest, and all were then seated on mats on the roof, behind low tables on which a great variety of delicacies had been placed. Next the head Lama handed to the winner a white scarf with three silver rupees, and to the second and third two and one rupee respectively, thus abolishing their amateur status at one stroke—being the thought that naturally occurred to my Western mind!

Next followed a horse race by the local village youths who unhitched their horses from their carriages and flung a leg over their backs with no saddle or cloth. The same course was set and the winners came to receive white scarves and prizes too.

It was now time for me to leave as I had to be back on my ship 300 odd miles away by next morning. I shook hands finally with Dhardoh Rimpoche and thanked him for his hospitality. By what great good fortune had I chanced to arrive on a day of a festival such as this!

Back on the ship things had suddenly changed and now I was to see the reason of all those questions asked by officers about our captain, especially as to whether we had any trouble with him. His personality had altered completely, even being reflected in his face. Now no longer jovial and paternal he wore a sullen discontented expression and his manner was aggressive and hostile. The difference was amazing.

Thereafter for the rest of the time I was on the ship we would alternate without warning between the two, and when in his second personality he would start pulling people up for doing what he had seen and allowed them to do for weeks past, all the time he had been his old, jolly self. No one knew where he was with him. For example, I had always gone ashore when work was finished and often I had met him as I was leaving with the bicycle and he would make some friendly crack about it. Now he suddenly sent for me one day on my return and demanded to know why I went ashore without asking his permission each time. Theoretically one should but many captains would not be bothered, and he had always been so friendly I had not done so since the last Captain of the *Bath* had told me not to bother him about it, but to go when I wanted if not going to be away for a night.

It was the same with the deck officers. One night apparently, he had not been able to sleep so he sent for the Second Mate in the morning to know why the bell was not being rung every half hour, why only for the change of watches. The answer was that it never had been. Technically again, it should be but there are few captains, much less passengers who would like their rest disturbed by it. Thereafter the officer of the watch banged it lustily every half hour. It was not his sleep that would be disturbed!

By the time we had reached the States again it was the most unhappy ship I had been on, after being the happiest. As there had been no passengers the Purser was out to save and the standard of meals deteriorated so much that there were constant complaints. Nor did we have any fresh fruit between India, the States and India again, although there was plenty available and he was supposed to buy fresh fruit and vegetables at the various ports, the frozen and tinned foods being in stock.

Naturally drinking became heavier and quarrels frequent. When the Captain was in his paternal personality he was perfectly approachable for the righting of abuses—usually connected with the food—but when he was in his second, it was unsafe to approach him at all.

We began the coasting voyage down America and there was still something to be had out of cycling ashore. Philadelphia and Boston, and Baltimore all fell before my wheel, and in these smaller places cycling seemed not so unusual as in New York; there were other cyclists about.

One Sunday with one of the apprentices who had the day off, I went to Washington by bus. We saw the White House, but no sign of Eisenhower, and we climbed the Washington Memorial [*sic*], some two thousand odd steps, up and down again, instead of going up in the lift, and then sank exhausted on some grassy verge to recover. Eventually we went to a drugstore and bought a banana split each [of] which was so monstrous that one between three would have been ample. However, having paid for them we considered it our duty to wade right through, which took quite a long time, but we managed it in the end!

One more trip I was to have ashore before the blow fell. The Mission to Seamen in Baltimore arranged an outing by bus for any seamen who wanted to go to Valley Forge, the scene of one of the epic wars of the War of Independence and both apprentices, myself and a Junior Engineer took advantage of this. The padre was a little man who had spent much time on missionary work in India and had known a lady passenger, a nurse missionary, we had taken out on the first trip, so she made a special point of giving us the history of the battle scene since our knowledge of that aspect of history was woefully small.

The log cabins were things as they were and to go inside one, and the house where Washington planned his last strategy and ate his last meal there could be seen just as he had left it.

We returned to the ship well pleased with our day's outing. And I went to sleep that night all unsuspecting of what was in store on the morrow.

As usual I was in the surgery shortly after eight o'clock to attend [those] of the crew who might need medicine, though often there would be none coming, when a steward brought me a cable. Wondering who on earth could be cabling from England and whether it was from Rampa whose exposure in the newspapers had filtered through by letters from friends, I opened it and read:

"Do you intend to claim the title since your change-over? Kindly cable *Daily Express*."

The reference to my change-over could only mean one thing, my secret had leaked out after *fifteen* years. Here was the end of my emancipation! But had Bobby died, which might account for the leakage? My hand trembled as I screwed the cable up and threw it in the wastepaper basket. Then along came the agent to tell me two reporters were wanting to see me and were in his office on the wharf. He gave no sign whether he knew why they were there.

There was nothing to be done except accept the inevitable. I went back to my cabin, lit my pipe to steady my nerves, and put on my cap without which one should not go ashore, and went down the gangway, my old poker face put aside, once more resumed.

The two reporters, one armed with a camera, were not unsympathetic, but they made it clear they had a job to do and were not to be diverted from it. And they wanted a photograph. If I did not consent they would take it anyway, so they might as well be allowed to get a good one. There was nothing for it but to sit there; puffing at my pipe and let them take it. Finally after answering questions in the shortest possible way and volunteering nothing, I was allowed to leave.

I made a bee-line for the Captain's cabin praying he might be in his paternal mood. He was pacing the deck in his shirt sleeves but went into his cabin and we sat down. I then told him about the reporters, that they were here solely on my private business, because it had somehow been discovered by the press that I was heir to a title and had "changed my sex," after the secret had been well kept for fifteen years.

He became kindly and sympathetic at once and promised to do all he could to help, which would consist chiefly in keeping reporters off the ship there and when we arrived in New York in a day or two, for we were sailing next day. He thereupon cabled the agents in New York asking for a police guard for the gangway.

Now I went into breakfast knowing I had about eight hours respite before the evening papers would be out and my brother officers would know. That morning I paced the upper deck struggling with myself: here was something for which Work Ideas were of paramount use and importance. "Nothing in life can hurt you if only you can learn not to react," I kept repeating over and over again to myself. But to repeat and to apply are two so different things. The upshot was that the intensity of the reaction was reduced by perhaps half of what it would have been as I tried every means of attention-distracting and mindfulness of anything I could find to do, to prevent its manifesting. Now would have been the time for some chipping and painting, but that avenue was closed. There was only reading or playing a game called Scrabble, which was in the lounge for passengers and which I had borrowed, to play with the apprentices who were not allowed in the lounge.

Next morning I knew they must all know but no one gave a sign. All the morning I sat in my cabin and no one came near me though I would have given anything for one or other officer to have dropped in for a drink or a casual chat. Only the Third Mate looked in once bouncing in his usual manner and saying:

"There's a photographer on the gangway, what would you like us to do with him?" Immensely grateful for this casual entrance, I grinned and showed him with a jerk of my thumb, and he laughed and went out again. He himself had been born with a hare-lip which had not been repaired until he was going to sea, and so he must have suffered much from the callousness of children at school.

At mealtimes everybody was studiously normal but the whole day passed without anyone coming near me. Even the apprentices seemed busy and I was not sure whether they knew or not, since none of the officers would have discussed it with anyone so low in the scale and they did not see the newspapers.

Next day I could stand it no longer and I took the bull by the horns and went up to the Second's cabin at twelve o'clock, the hour for drinks and social converse. He and Sparks were in there and I was at once invited in for a drink. I made a direct attack by asking if they had seen the papers and what was their attitude going to be. The Second poured me out a gin, raised his glass and knocked mine and then said that they had discussed it at length over beer the night before and had come to the conclusion that I had had a raw deal and since they had liked me before and I had not changed overnight they saw no reason for letting it make any difference.

I went down to lunch with a much lighter heart. But I had also learned that only a single officer was inimical, and that was the Mate as one might have expected. He was saying of course he always had felt something was wrong but couldn't put a finger on it and now it was obvious. But he got no support in this. He was also saying with a sneer with reference to the photo which had been published in the *Baltimore Sun*, how I had sat for it especially.

Next morning he and I were alone at breakfast and I asked him:
"Have you ever been in the hands of the press?"
"No," he said with a smirk.

"Then don't judge too harshly, before you have," I said. "Those reporters told me they would take a photograph with or without my permission;
otherwise there would have been none."

He continued eating in silence. How I longed for Jack or Willie at this
time. How different would such a period of trial have been. But then . . .
"those circumstances in which you find yourself are the best for you to
work on" and "whatever the circumstances if you take them as work, you
will come out unbroken." Anyway the Irish in me would never permit
of my giving way under any circumstances whatsoever. But I could have
wished to have been spared these.

We reached New York where we lay for ten days loading. The agent
came on, all sympathy and told me of the arrangements that had been made
for my protection, a company's servant and a policeman on the gangway
but on no account to try and go ashore since the police themselves had said
they could not then offer adequate protection; the photographers would
try and tear the clothes off me to get a picture. Such is the state of modern
civilization, so progressive as it is believed to be. Then he added:

"You *are* the working doctor, aren't you? Didn't I see you down the
hatches last time you were here?"

I admitted it with a wry grin and added that with this Mate it was no
longer possible, at which he nodded and then left.

For those ten days I was confined not only to the ship but to its starboard deck, that one away from the wharf. The first morning there I had
gone out on the upper deck and looked down and the wharf was filled with
milling people, many waving cameras. I shot across the deck to the other
side and there made my morning promenade daily, without my coat for the
weather was warm, my hands dug deep into my trousers' pockets and my
black tie fluttering in the breeze. Up and down, up and down.

What to do now was the question. I could never set foot ashore in America with safety again. Probably the company would allow me to change
ships in India, but then if I arrived back in England would my advent be
heralded and reporters once more be waiting? As yet I had no information
as to how this had come about.

Then from G. came a letter and a copy of the *Sunday Express*, which he
had been wont to send periodically anyway. Page three, under Ephraim
Hardcastle's social column was the Headline: *Strange Case of Dr. Dillon*.
Then two columns were spent explaining that a discrepancy had been
found between Burke and Debrett about the heir to the title of baronetcy
after Sir Robert Dillon the present holder. It added that all attempts to

get Sir Robert to say where his sister was working or what she was doing had been to no avail. A doctor somewhere in England, was all he would say.

How Bobby must have hated and feared those reporters! Small wonder that it seems as if on the second day he broke down and gave away the name of my ship; then it was only a matter of consulting Lloyd's register to find out where she was. A further newspaper cutting gave the history of my having changed from a lady doctor into a naval surgeon quite erroneously, since I had never been a lady doctor, but most of their facts were inaccurate.

Letters started coming now from my oldest friends, offering their sympathy and saying what they thought of the press. Sir Harold Gillies also wrote, and the Lady Warden from the Mission to Seamen, and, of course, Lobzang Rampa, who himself had been in the papers in the past two months. One and all they wrote encouragement.

Then I sat down and composed a letter to Ellerman Lines apologizing for having all unwittingly involved them in my unexpected publicity and I had two letters back, one from the Chairman to offer his sympathy and another from the Medical Superintendent saying he "still hoped I would stay with the company and would back any arrangements I liked." But it would have been an impossible situation, boarding any new ship I would have been the target for speculation and whispers, until they got to know me and it was too much for me to whom release from being a museum piece had come as so great a boon.

I also wrote to my London Club which I had joined some years before with the aide of a passenger who had put me up for it, since it was a large and well known one and tendered my resignation saying that I imagined they would not wish me to remain a member. In due course a letter came back from the Secretary to say the committee had considered my letter and had decided to refuse my resignation since there was no blame to be attached to me in the matter but please not mention the Club's name to the press. I thereupon sent them a cheque for a two year's overseas subscription and said I would be away for that length of time.

For now was being born the idea of asking for my discharge from the ship in India and setting about not only disappearing but finding a monastery. Dhardoh Rimpoche having given me his Kalimpong address before I left and told me to come and see him there when I was free, I imagined he might take me in to his monastery, not knowing then that he had none in Kalimpong.

I wrote again to the Medical Superintendent of the company and asked for my release in Calcutta as I could not go back to the States and it would not be safe to return to England yet. I thought to disappear in India for a while till all the fuss had died down. And to this he consented. The ship did not carry over a hundred personnel and could sail back to the States without me. He would arrange with the Calcutta agents.

One more letter I wrote other than those to friends; and this was to the editor of the *Sunday Express*, asking him whether he had stopped to think before publishing what might be the effect on a doctor's career of such a denouement. Since I had committed no crime and was undeserving of publicity, what justification had he? And I enclosed a defensive article entitled *A Ship's Surgeon Speaks*, for publication, putting right many of the printed errors and calling for a better sense of values.

Needless to say it was not printed. It came back along with a nice letter from the editor saying he had been deeply moved by letter and article, but he thought it best not to publish the letter since it would only mean more publicity and his justification was that he had a duty to the public.

It was gratifying to see that only a few weeks later he was arraigned before the press commission for having pursued the family of an executed murderer across the world and had reporters waiting on the quayside when the ship that was to have carried them to a new life elsewhere reached its destination, so that their story was immediately known to those among whom they had hoped to be able to start afresh without prejudice or knowledge. Again he had pleaded his duty to the public. The plea was rejected, and I reject it in my own case. It was a most heartless piece of interference in an individual's private concerns.

But now there was much to be done if my plans were to be put into effect. When I first told the Captain I had asked for my release in Calcutta he had nodded kindly and said that was all right, he was very sorry about it all. Only later was he to rescind this due to his second personality. This second personality was always looking for some grounds for resentment, which was why he would suddenly attack a practice he had previously condoned, and it reveled in self pity, which was forgotten again when he became his old self. The prospect of my leaving the ship was thus picked upon as a source of grievance after a week or so out from America. He, the Captain, would have to do the surgery on top of all his own work. But in the Ellerman Lines the Purser always did it and not the Captain when there was no surgeon on board. It was no use telling him that, he would have to do it and I was the cause of it. Having a grievance kept him in his second personality much longer periods at a time and before I left it was almost his permanent one.

From the moment I had decided to go ashore and look for a monastery I set about preparing myself for it without knowing much about conditions in monasteries, beyond what I had seen at Bodh Gaya.

Firstly I would certainly have to get used to sitting cross-legged which I had not done since school days. Trying for the first time my knees were high up in the air and just would not go down! It was also a painful position for my tightened ligaments and stiffened joints. I sat down on the carpet and took my watch off and put it on the deck in front of me. There I would sit for a quarter of an hour and there I did sit for a quarter of an hour. The first five minutes was not too bad, the second I was wanting to uncurl and the third was sheer agony. Only by grimly refusing to relax did I stay there and then had to undo my knees with my hands.

Daily this went on, every evening before supper. Then as it became easier I bethought me of that game of Scrabble. If I sat on my settee and played with myself, right hand against left, the game took about three quarters of an hour to complete and was after the nature of a crossword puzzle, then my mind being distracted I might be able to stay the period. So every afternoon after lunch I began to play Scrabble sitting cross-legged on the settee. By the time we had reached India I could stay those three quarters of an hour fairly comfortably and my knees had come down quite a long way although still not flat out.

Perhaps also one might have to kneel for long periods. I did not know. But to be on the safe side I practiced that too, although my creaking joints protested, and also tried bending backwards to lie between my feet when in a kneeling position, and did various other exercises designed to loosen up tightened ligaments in thighs and knees.

Then there was the matter of meditation. All I knew about that was that it involved concentration and stopping the teeming thoughts. Lying on my bunk one hot day in only my shorts it occurred to me that if one watched one's abdomen rising and falling as one breathed this might be a focus of concentration and help control the mind. All unknowingly I had hit upon the method used in Burma called the *Vissipassana Method* [sic], about which much has been written by its adherents, although it is criticized in other schools of meditation as being faulty.

But it never occurred to me to study Buddhism at all or to look for books on it when we were in Bombay or Colombo. I had no ideas about changing my religion whatsoever.

A dock strike was in progress in Bombay and we lay at anchor outside the harbor for ten days waiting for a berth and one day could count sixty two ships lying around us. When we did enter port it was a relief to find that my story had not penetrated to the Indian papers, and I could go about with all my old confidence unafraid of curious stares and whispers.

But there was an unpleasant task to be performed. If I were to go ashore in Calcutta all my unnecessary gear would have to go back to England in one of the company's ships. But the bicycle must be sold, the faithful old blue and white bicycle which had accompanied me in so many countries of the world from the Far West to the Far East. It was no use sending that to be damaged en route and lie rusting till I was to come again.

Feeling like a murderer I mounted it for the last time at the foot of the gangway and rode slowly out of the dock gates to find a cycle dealer. Seventy rupees or about £5 was all they would give, despite the three speed gear and as I left I turned and saw it being wheeled away seemingly to death, reproaching me for handing it over to strangers thus. Later I was to write a short story entitled "The Bicycle" which the *Sunday Statesman* published and paid ninety rupees for and the main hero of it was the same blue and white bicycle I had so callously left behind in Bombay.

On board it was time to start settling my affairs, which entailed writing to my usual correspondents and telling them of my intention to disappear for a couple of years and to return to England in 1961. Meanwhile please would no one try and find out where I was or write until I wrote first. They all wrote back sad at the temporary parting but understanding of the situation. G. was especially upset but still was hopeful that it would not be too long before we met again. Meanwhile I sent him a cheque to cover his son's school fees for another year and assured him they would never be forgotten.

Calcutta came at last. My payoff for these eight months on board less all withdrawals would come to about two hundred pounds, and on this I intended to live without recourse to money from England. In a monastery one would not have much chance of spending, one would think.

The agents told me it was necessary to take a plane to Chittagong and back again because I had entered India as a seaman and they would be held responsible for me until I reentered it as a tourist. This would be a waste of money but a seeming necessity and inescapable.

On my last night on board, all my uniform and unwanted goods packed and only a zip bag left to take with me, I had a warm bath and as I lay in it I wondered when the next one like that would be for I had no illusions as to the possible hardship there might be in store. Indeed I had been sleeping out on the deck with only a blanket beneath me when other officers brought out their mattresses, in anticipation of a hard bed to come.

Now I climbed into my bunk for the last time and lay there thinking of these past six years at sea. On the whole they had been good with the exception of this last voyage. Yet, had it been a happy ship the parting might have been much harder. As it was there would be few regrets at leaving her. One of the apprentices was to be transferred to a home-going ship and there was no sign of captain or Mate being shifted. And the food had remained poor although since America I had withheld any further complaints thinking, rightly as it turned out, that probably shortly I would look back on these meals as luxurious compared with what might be in store for me.

I recalled the day I joined my first ship, my premature baby, and my unhappiness in Hong Kong. And many things, too, not listed in this narrative as they would have taken too long. There was the trip to Malacca by bus from Singapore and the strange event on the way; my visit to Macao by ferry from Hong Kong and another to the borders of Red China behind Kowloon with the assistant commissioner of police and a sight of Red soldiers, with tommy guns at the ready on their side of the barbed wire, while a British policeman, revolver in holster strolled nonchalantly on his side. Meeting my cousin Joan in Tanga and again in Aden and the dance we went to at the club there. Las Palmas with its continental cafes and beautiful trees, of the Captains I had sailed with and the Mates who had taught me to work the ship . . .

But all this was now the past and must be forgotten. It was the future which was important, completely in the dark as it was. Would Dhardoh Rimpoche remember and take me into his monastery? That was what I was expecting, hoping. To get away from the world for a while and fit myself for coping with it better. All this time had been but a preparation for that future. There was nothing that had not played its part, even that which had given me such ample opportunity for the practice of Gurdjieffian ideas. Had I never met them, how different might everything have been and how much more would I have suffered! Suicide is the answer others like myself have sometimes found. But suicide is no answer though one may feel like it.

There is nothing for man in this world but conquest of his mind; of the way he takes the world in all its absurdities and pompous imaginings. What is it the Work teaches?

"Remember the whole secret is, in this Teaching, not to try to change external circumstances, because if you do not change yourself and the way you take the repeating events of life, everything will recur in the same way. As long as you remain as you are in yourself you will attract the same problems, same difficulties, same situation but if you change yourself your life will change." And, "You cannot reform the world; you can only reform your way of taking in the world."

CHAPTER 13

Imji Getsul

Those who have read *Imji Getsul* which told of my experiences while serving in a Ladakh monastery as a novice-monk will perceive that in the second chapter thereof, which the publishers demanded should be inserted because they wanted to know how I ever came to be a Buddhist monk at all, there have been slight twists to the story to mislead those who had known me in England who were close friends, so that idle chatter as to my possible identity would not reach the ears of the press and send reporters flying out to my haven of refuge.

Thus my unique combination of degrees, known to many, might have served as a clue, for who else had read Greats at Oxford and then added medical degrees to it? Also since my previous denouement occurred when I was serving as surgeon in the Merchant Navy, this also might have touched a chord, hence I gave the impression that I had signed on as a deck hand, stretching the emphasis on my hobby at sea a little far, perhaps. *Mutatis mutandis . . .*

And now I was on the plane to Siliguri, the nearest airfield to Kalimpong, yet still fifty miles away, with Dhardoh Rimpoche's card in my breast pocket. From Siliguri we had to go by "bus" or by what passed by the courtesy title of "bus," a truck, to our destination and when we arrived it was four in the afternoon and a thunderstorm was in progress. A taxi took me on and left me on the main road, the driver having pointed down the mountain to what looked like a country house set in fields and had said the Lama lived there.

How was I to know what had been happening in those months at sea? It seemed there had been a French ex–Roman Catholic nun who had persuaded Rimpoche against his judgment to make her a Buddhist nun or getsulma. Thereafter she had caused havoc in the area for she was keenly obsessed by sex repressions and had started bringing all sorts of charges against various Sikkimese and Bhutanese monks and Lamas as well as influential laymen. She was also being used by certain Communist agents to obtain information about these areas. The rest of her story is outside the scope of this one; it is well known to all in India since finally questions were asked about her in the Lok Sabha and Mr. Nehru had put an end to all things by saying he understood that she was a little unbalanced.* Finally she went back to France and proceeded to write a book against Buddhism, so it is said.

All unaware of the fear of Westerners that this had produced in the minds of Tibetan and Sikkimese Lamas, I arrived on the doorstep of Dhardoh Rimpoche's house, tired and hungry, for I had not slept the night before from mosquitos at the Seamen's Club and had not eaten since breakfast.

He would not see me, but sent a message that he was ill. I sat down on my bag, utterly weary with my hopes blasted, and even the tea and biscuits he sent down by his monk attendant did nothing to revive me.

What was I to do now? I sat on, thinking perhaps this might be one of those tests Gurus were wont to put to prospective disciples to see if they had stamina and determination. But nothing happened. At length his attendant came and said he had been told to take me to the English bhikshu of Kalimpong, and the stalwart monk shouldered my heavy bag, still containing the Viewmaster and a large set of pictures I had bought as a present for my intended Guru.

We took a taxi some way and then were decanted once more above a mountain path and the monk heaved up the bag and set off down the steep

* The Lok Sabha is the Indian Parliament. Jawaharlal Nehru was the first prime minister of India, serving first as the head of the interim government after independence from Britain, then as elected head of the new state after partition from 1947 to 1964.

slope at a pace with which my tired feet, stumbling on loose stones, would not keep up. Despondency had added to my weariness.

He turned off down a little garden path where there was a red roof house and put my bag down on the verandah. Sitting inside a large room was a young man dressed in a yellow robe with his right shoulder bare and he looked up with some annoyance at the interruption.

The monk spoke to him in Hindi and he beckoned me to come in. This was the beginning of my stay at a vihara, the Hindi word for a monastery, for the next four months. That same night I told the bhikshu why I had come and of the events that had led up to my sudden unexpected arrival, since, being a monastery, and not knowing whether my publicity would follow me there, I did not wish him to be entertaining what he knew not. He, on his side, assured me that anything I told him would be as if under the seal of the confessional, or as a medical confidence, and I trusted him because he was both a fellow Englishman and a monk. How misplaced that trust was I could not foresee. Before going to bed I threw my pipe down the cliff knowing it would be of no benefit for me in the monasteries.

There was no idea in my mind at this time of becoming a Buddhist knowing nothing about that religion and being satisfied with what Christ had taught if not with the way the Church had distorted it. But I wanted to read some more about it since Lin Yu Tung's book had been a promising beginning. Meanwhile I paid five rupees a day for my keep and readily typed for my host and worked in the garden for exercise. He was writing his own autobiography then, and there was plenty of typing to be done.

It was a beautiful spot, on top of a mountain two miles out of Kalimpong, and from the verandah you could look across the Teesta Valley to the mountains behind which Darjeeling was situated, and far below the Teesta river wound, frothing its way over rocks in its narrow bed. To the right was Kunchenjunga, famous Mountain of Snow above which the rising sun would slowly appear, a great crimson ball, shedding its pink glow on the snowy caps, and to the left were the flanks of mountains on which were dotted small homesteads, farming plots of land in terraced fashion even as our own garden was terraced down the cliff.

Beside the main building which had been a bungalow and had been kindly presented to the bhikshu by a well known author and traveled there was an annex consisting of four rooms, about eight feet by six, supposed to be for monks. Here I was put to sleep on a wooden bed, which is the Indian counterpart of a spring mattress, and showed the wise foresight in my preliminary practice of sleeping on deck. There was a Pali puja or form of temple service morning and evening at six o'clock, and it was followed by meditation for as long as the bhikshu himself remained in it, maybe half an hour maybe an hour.

I was happy for it was peaceful and after a few days we went down to visit Dhardoh Rimpoche and to give him his Viewmaster, and he decided that this was the best arrangement that could be made. It was then that I learned of the French nun whom I was later to meet.

For four months I stayed and worked daily, and learned the Pali puja by heart so that I could join in. Once a month we had a public puja to which surrounding Buddhists came, few as they were, but perhaps half a dozen Western ones. My name I had requested should not be revealed and the bhikshu gave me the name of Jivaka, after the Buddha's physician in the Pali canon. (At first I was impressed by his mature calm manner and thought to take him for my guru.)

But he would not teach me, thirsting though I was for all the knowledge I could acquire. "No, you learn too fast," he said. This was true. I have an odd facility for picking up a subject quickly but that should surely be a reason for teaching and not for refraining. Sometimes if someone came to call, tourists or acquaintances, I would listen outside the door to try and glean something. For he was good at explaining when he wanted to, but he volunteered nothing whatsoever and only selected special books out of his library for me to read instead of giving me the run of it.

Sometimes a Tibetan Lama would come but he did not encourage any contact between him and myself. Then came time for his winter tour when he would go out preaching to the "new" Buddhists (convertees among the peasantry due to the late Dr. Ambedkar's movement), for he was a very good preacher. He decided that he would take me to Sarnath, a place I had never heard of, and leave me there as there was a pilgrim's Dharmasala or Rest-House there where I could stay free and only have to provide my own food. He would be away three months.

This was the beginning of my real interest in Buddhism for, apart from the bhikshus there, there was a library of some size, in which were many of the English translations of the Pali canon by the London Pali Text Society and now I could read without restriction. Meanwhile every morning at five o'clock I would go over to the great Mulagandhakuti Vihara or Sinhalese Temple and practice meditation for an hour.

Before he returned I had completed my first book, called *Practicing the Dharmapada*, taking twenty texts out of this traditional first book for followers of the Buddha and writing an essay on them, strongly Gurdjieffian in flavor for by now it was obvious that Gurdjieff had drawn very largely on Buddhism *inter alia*. Unfortunately the book was still-born for it was even worse printed than most Indian productions which seem incapable of matching the works of other countries.

All available of the Pali canon I read and some Western scholars' works on the history and philosophy of Buddhism and within three months I saw in the world renunciation of the Buddhist monk a way in keeping with my sense of values which rated the pleasures of the world very low. Money making for its own sake had never appealed to me, nor had luxurious living. And hence on the bhikshu's return I received the Lower Ordination of the sramanera or novice-monk of the Theravadin Order, which is the Hinayana School or Sect of Buddhism. For at that time I knew little more than the name of the rival Sect nor did I know how bigoted and intolerant were the Theravadins towards their Northern brethren.

World renunciation means renunciation of the things of the world. I set about making my "will" and communicated with my solicitor and stockbroker, as the tale has been told before in *Imji Getsul*, and disposed of all my property, not forgetting the Mission to Seamen in Victoria Dock Road for all the good work it does.

Then I went back to Kalimpong with the bhikshu and gave him, as being my Guru, presumably, since I was living with him, all the remains of my pay-off, or about £130 and my automatic watch and gold signet ring to sell. This last was a marked wrench, which was why I made myself part with it. Despite other values being different, this one worldly value still had some hold on me and even now I think of the ring wistfully, and despise myself for so doing.

But the peace and happiness that had seemed to be in the vihara now did not last and within three months I left the bhikshu. He had a large number of Hindu youths whom he called his "students" although only to a few of them did he teach English. In that part of India on the borders of Nepal family life is strict and sons dare not even speak to their fathers, so that many of them were only too glad to get away from parental control and live at the vihara while attending school each day. For in India youths of over twenty may still be at school. And equally there parents were only too glad to be rid of the trouble and cost of having them at home if someone could be found who was so foolish as to take them in.

They played him for a sucker and he fondly imagined himself as their father. Even one of the elder and nicer ones told me he was had, they only liked him for what they could get out of him, but he had convinced himself that they were all his family. It was this that led to my departure.

When he had no money he could not afford to have them there except occasionally, but now that he had had a sudden lump sum within weeks the vihara had acquired five youths all living on the bhikshu (two of their fathers paid one rupee a day for their keep) and being outside any monastic discipline they were rude and noisy. My room was no longer a quiet haven for next door two boys shared a room and talked and laughed and read out of the newspaper when I was trying to work or meditate. When I complained the bhikshu suggested my working somewhere else. I pointed out that it was I who was the monk, not they, and they should be asked to be quiet in a vihara, but to no avail. They could do no wrong, everyone must be subservient to them.

It was now that having finished *Growing Up Into Buddhism*, written for teenagers, I was working on my popular version of the *Life of Milarepa*, which has just been published, to make a racy story out of the rather too learned and academic one of Evans-Wentz, so as to bring it to the notice of the public, for the story itself is attractive enough for it to be a world-wide classic and not merely a Tibetan one.

But in addition to the noise another factor was prominent. Very quickly the money disappeared and food became scarce with so many mouths to feed. From ship meals I had in any case been precipitated suddenly in middle life into a vegetarian diet of rice and curried vegetables and, not having the distended stomach of the rice eater from birth, I was hard put to get enough to eat, since after but a little rice I would suffer from uncomfortable distension and within half an hour would be ravenously hungry again. But up to now there had been an egg provided each day at breakfast for the ex-meat eaters, and this applied to all the youths too who were not naturally vegetarian.

With so many to feed first the eggs gave out and then the butter, and there came one morning when there were only two small slices of dry bread for breakfast for each person, because there was no money left. What he had done with it all I do not know, but he would always give it to the boys if they asked to borrow some. That day I went up to an English lady, wife of a Sikkimese landowner, living a mile away and begged for some breakfast. It could not go on. Still untaught, now also unfed and with no quietness, there was nothing to stay for. I would go back to Sarnath, though how to live would be a problem. The bhikshu, not at all averse to being left alone with his boys, agreed and set about raising the money for my fare and when he had it I departed.

We were still on friendly terms but there was a matter which was going to prove a problem. The first thing noticeable in reading the Buddhist canon is the casual reference not to two but to the three sexes, and there are many bans on various types of people from receiving the Higher Ordination, among them being anyone belonging to this "third sex." Others are all those who have suffered any form of mutilation, loss of eye or nose or hand or foot, of being lame, etc., and with various diseases all bringing them under the ban. The reason was that in the Buddha's day such people were probably criminals who had received judicial punishment in terms of amputation, as is still done in the Middle East today, and someone with a criminal record is not a good candidate for the monkhood. Also in the Buddha's day the monks lived often in the jungle and had to walk through it on their begging rounds, and so it was a necessity to be able bodied. But today when war or traffic accidents and not crime produces mutilations, the reason for the ban had gone and the upholding of it in many cases might be a gross injustice to a worthy individual. But the keynote of Theravadin or Hinayana Buddhism is adherence to the letter of the law. The spirit is secondary. Whereas in Mahayana Buddhism it is the spirit that counts and the letter can be altered within the spirit. The spirit of the bans is to exclude undesirable people from the *sangha* or Monkhood. If a bodily defect is not accompanied by a mental or spiritual defect it is not regarded as requiring to be upheld as a ban. But the person may be tested the more severely first to see if he really is in his heart a true monk. And this is in accordance with the Buddha's Compassion for He, Himself, whenever He is said to have made a rule, if it was brought to his notice that the keeping of the rule would necessitate undue hardship or even death in certain cases he always modified it immediately.

I was anxious for Higher Ordination and had found all this in my reading. When I asked the bhikshu about the prospects of it he said in contemptuous tones:

"Oh yes, in three or four years perhaps."

The contempt in his voice made me wonder. Slowly, slowly and unwillingly I began to think his refusal to teach me and studied indifference might be due to its being a case of "Bears like a Turk no brother near the throne."

Then came the time in Sarnath, after some months when one of the bhikshus there offered to give me the Higher Ordination and make me a bhikshu. At once I told him it was not easy as I came under one of the bans and I even mentioned which. So for the present the matter was dropped.

Meanwhile Tibetan Lamas had been visiting Sarnath and I had met many while living next door. One [was] Lochas Rimpoche, who was being kept by a Ladakhi monk in charge of seventeen small Ladakhi boys who were being educated in Sarnath. (He appears in greater detail in *Imji Getsul*.) Lochas Rimpoche was destitute although he had been a Professor of Philosophy in Drespung and was highly thought of among his own people as a scholar. Their behavior appealed to me much more than that of the Theravadin bhikshu who thinks himself superior to everyone else except senior bhikshus, and I began to lean toward the Mahayana Sect and wondered if it were possible to be ordained by them. But here language was the difficulty. At that time Lama Lobzang's English was very restricted and Lochas Rimpoche had none.

He agreed to ordain me so I wrote to the English bhikshu asking him if he would like to come to Sarnath for it, and wondering what I could do about explaining things in view of the language problem.

He did not reply, or the letter never arrived, and I suddenly thought of a Kulu layman who was at the Sanskrit University in Varanasi who spoke quite good English as well as Tibetan and to him I went with the problem and told him all about myself. He promised to come over the next Sunday to explain to Lochas Rimpoche and see if there was any objection to my ordination in the Tibetan way of thinking.

Before this could happen to my horror on the Saturday morning I was shown a letter by the bhikshu to whom I had first confided, in which the English bhikshu had given away all my confidences and added a few more imaginary details of his own. What was more this letter had been sent out in triplicate to the Chief bhikshu of Sarnath and to Lama Lobzang. The latter up to that time had fairly worshipped the English bhikshu and he was completely shattered by his action. He [the English bhikshu] subsequently defended his action by saying it was his *duty*, in order to protect the *sangha* and monkhood (and he could easily have stayed my ordination with no more than a hint). In fact he was furious that I should receive full ordination so quickly (actually there is no time limit set) so that he betrayed everything I had so unwisely told him and then added that of course he would never tell a layman a word about it.

Naturally everything was off for the moment.

"It's a very small matter really," Lochas Rimpoche had said, so Lama Lobzang told me, "but since so much noise has been made about it we can't do anything just now."

Shortly after this His Holiness the Dalai Lama came to stay in Sarnath for a month, again this visit has already been described in my other book. Suffice it to say that I asked Lama Lobzang to tell the whole story to the Dalai Lama's Senior Guru who was there and have a verdict from him, so one afternoon we went down to see him and found Kushok Bakula, Head Lama of Ladakh and later to become my chief Guru, there too. Both were told, and Kushok gave me a look of compassion which I will never forget. Both said it was not impossible for me to be ordained fully, but to wait till the noise had died down. Having already taken the Bodhisattva Vow from the Senior Guru, let that suffice for the present.

Instead, as readers of *Imji Getsul* know, I was reordained as a novice-monk, by Lochas Rimpoche, to be called in the future a getsul and not a sramanera, and to have Lobzang added to my Pali name which could not be changed because I had become quite well known in Buddhist journals for my writings already. I am the first foreigner the Tibetans have ordained.

Then when I went to Rizong Monastery in Ladakh, Kushok Bakula promised me he would give me the Higher Ordination on my return the following year. Here other factors intervened.

In India there is a marked phobia of imperialist spies, although none such exist at any rate from among Westerners. I had begun writing for the *Hindustan Times Sunday Weekly* on Tibetan Buddhism and over the first article the editor wanted a snippet of autobiography in which I mentioned I had been to a Ladakh monastery the last years and hoped to return that year. A Communist weekly paper called the *Blitz* had seized on this and written a column on me charging me with being in the British Intelligence, an ex–Royal Naval officer and a spy especially hired by Mr. Nehru to spy on the Chinese in Ladakh.

The fantastic-ness of this was so great that it never occurred to me any-one would believe it. But they did! Eventually two Communist M.P.'s asked questions in the Lok Sabha about my visit to the defense area of Ladakh and Mr. Nehru vigorously defended me, saying I was a genuine Buddhist and not merely "posing" as a monk as they had said.

But there was no further permit given, hard though I tried to obtain one. Further there suddenly appeared, some months later, in a local Hindi newspaper some story of my having once been a lady-doctor who had changed her sex and had now become a Buddhist monk. Where it came from I do not know. Rumor pinned it on a Sarnath Indian bhikshu but he denied it. Anyway the fact remained that they had been talking and it had leaked out. Fortunately no one takes any notice what is in Hindi lo-cal rags and it was not taken up elsewhere. In fact the English language papers would have been most embarrassed by it since it would mean that all their allegations about being a spy and a Royal Naval officer must be wrong.

Final handwritten note: "This chapter is tentative and depends on whether things finally come out due to the English bhikshu or otherwise. [Illegible: perhaps "If they do"] from him the further story of his writing to Christmas Humphreys the leading editor of the *Middle Way* can be added. Anyway if you think the whole subject better omitted it can be too. I can leave off at where I reach Kalimpong."

July 28, 1914	World War I begins in Europe
May 1, 1915	Laura Maude Dillon born in Ladbroke Grove, London
May 11, 1915	Dillon's mother, Laura Maude (Reese), dies from sepsis. Dillon and older brother Robert are brought to live with their father's maiden sisters in Folkestone.
November 11, 1918	Armistice Day, conclusion of World War I
October 6, 1925	Dillon's father, Robert, dies of pneumonia, complicated by alcoholism
1930	Lili Elbe, who had been assigned male at birth, undergoes several transition-related surgeries which are reported in Danish and German newspapers. Elbe's marriage is declared invalid. She is able to change her name legally and to obtain a new passport.
1931	Death of Lili Elbe from surgical complications
1933	*Man Into Woman: An Authentic Record of a Change of Sex*, published by Niels Hoyer, the pseudonymous name of E. L. H. Jacobson. It narrates the story of Lili Elbe.
Fall 1934	Dillon starts at the Society of Home-Students, Oxford (now called St. Anne's College), switches out of Theology to Greats, and takes up rowing.
1935–1937	Dillon, now a stroke rower, Rowing Blue, is elected president of the Oxford University Women's Boat Club. Remains president until graduation. Is photographed by the *Daily Mirror* with the caption "Man or Woman?"
1935	Testosterone synthesized
1938	Dillon graduates, leaves Oxford

1939	World War II begins
	Dillon employed at a laboratory in Gloucestershire, working on brain research
	Seeks treatment for gender dysphoria, begins testosterone
	Begins working on the book that would become *Self: A Study in Ethics and Endocrinology*
November 24, 1940	first German blitz on Bristol
November 25, 1940	Dillon begins to work at a Bristol gas station; begins firewatching
April–July 1942	Baedeker Blitzes
June 27, 1942	Baedeker Blitz on Weston-super-Mare unfolds while Dillon is in the hospital there, recovering from a hypoglycemic blackout and fall
Late 1942 or early 1943	Dillon's double mastectomy
April 14, 1944	reregistration as Laurence Michael Dillon
October 30, 1944	Robert Allen, assigned female at birth, is reregistered under his male name
1945	World War II ends
	Dillon undergoes the first of thirteen operations for phalloplasty
Fall 1945	Dillon begins medical school at Trinity College, Dublin
1946	Dillon's *Self: A Study in Ethics and Endocrinology* is published by Butterworth-Heinemann
1947–1950	Portion of the Eastern British Indian Empire separates into India and Pakistan; both countries become independent. Jawaharlal Nehru elected prime minister of India.
1949	Dillon undergoes the last of his phalloplasty operations
1950	Dillon falls in love with Roberta Cowell
1950–1951	China invades Tibet
May 17, 1951	Roberta Cowell is officially reregistered under her female name
May/June 1951	Dillon completes medical school at Trinity College, Dublin, and takes a job at a small hospital north of Dublin. He begins reading the works of G. I. Gurdjieff and P. D. Ouspensky.

1952	Dillon joins the Merchant Navy as a ship's surgeon and begins traveling around the world. He begins avidly studying Ouspensky and Gurdjieff through Maurice Nicoll's *Psychological Commentaries.*
December 1, 1952	Christine Jorgensen's transition is announced in the press
June 2, 1953	Coronation of Elizabeth II as monarch of the British Empire
1954	*Roberta Cowell's Story* is published by British Book Center, Inc. *But for the Grace: The True Story of a Dual Existence* by Robert Allen is published by W. H. Allen. Allen emphasizes that his transition entailed no medical interventions.
December 1956	The Suez Crisis: Israel, Britain, and France invade Egypt in an attempt to remove Egyptian president Gamal Nasser from power and regain control of the Suez Canal. Britain grounds Merchant Navy ships, including Dillon's *City of Oxford*, until they are forced to withdraw by the United Nations.
1957	While in England between ships, Dillon publishes *Poems of Truth* through Linden Press and meets Lobzang Rampa, author of *The Third Eye*
May 1958	Newspapers worldwide report Dillon's history of transition throughout the month
Summer 1958	Dillon arrives in India, begins living in Sangharakshita's community in Kalimpong, the Triyana Vardhana Vihara. Given the name Jivaka by Sangharakshita Begins serious study of Buddhism
1959	Jivaka begins writing articles on Buddhism for English-speaking audiences March 2 ordained a *sramanera*, or novice monk, at Saranath Jivaka's *Practicing the Dhammapada* published by Maha Bodhi Press
End of 1959	Sangharakshita sends letters blocking Jivaka's *bhikshu* ordination

1960	Jivaka reordained a *getsul*, or novice monk, in the Tibetan Buddhist tradition
	Growing Up Into Buddhism, a book for youth, published by Maha Bodhi Press
	A Critical Study of the Vinaya published by Maha Bodhi Press
July–October 1960	Jivaka lives in Rizong Monastery in Ladakh
Winter 1960–1961	Jivaka ill in the hospital
Spring 1961	Jivaka accused of being an imperialist spy by the *Blitz*. Nehru defends him in front of Indian Parliament. Jivaka's visa permit is not renewed.
April 1962	*Life of Milarepa* published by John Murray (Wisdom of the East Series)
	Imji Getsul published by Routledge and Kegan Paul
May 15, 1962	Lobzang Jivaka dies in Dalhousie, India, while on his way to Kashmir

ACKNOWLEDGMENTS

This project has been a work of affection and endurance. It was first sparked in the spring of 2007 when we stood in the back of the Brookline Booksmith listening to Pagan Kennedy read from *The First Man-Made Man*, her biography of Michael Dillon/Lobzang Jivaka. Having come across a review of it in the *Boston Globe*, we were curious to learn more about this relatively unknown trans forebear who had not only transitioned during World War II but had also been a medical doctor and a Buddhist monastic novice before his sudden death. As students of both trans and religious studies, and as trans men ourselves, the evident intersection of these fields in Dillon/Jivaka's life were of particular interest. When Kennedy mentioned the unpublished memoir *Out of the Ordinary*, a key source both for her and for Liz Hodgkinson's biography *Michael née Laura*, we were keen to learn where to find it. How might the memoir become available to scholars and community members? When we approached Kennedy with these questions, she very kindly connected us to Andrew Hewson, the literary executor of the Dillon estate, and to the memoir itself. Reading it, we resolved to help fulfill Dillon/Jivaka's strong wish that it be published. Without Kennedy's encouragement and generosity and Hewson's supportive and patient willingness to work with us, this project would never have come to fruition.

In the twists and turns of the ensuing nine years, other projects, both professional and personal, coincided with and outpaced this one at several points. During this time we benefited from the wisdom, enthusiasm, and critique of numerous colleagues and friends. Cameron deeply appreciates the feedback he received on the project in Mark Jordan's Religion and Sexuality seminar at Emory University in 2010. He values the support and encouragement he has received from colleagues and students at the Divinity School and the Committee on Studies of Women, Gender, and Sexuality at Harvard University, as well as at Boston University and Episcopal Divinity School. When this project began, Cameron was completing his dissertation, had only recently begun ordained life as an Episcopal priest, and was not yet a dad. He especially thanks his spouse, Kateri, for her support and understanding during the late nights and time away that bringing this project to completion has required.

So many members of UCLA's Gender Studies Department have been invaluable in the process of seeing Dillon/Jivaka's memoir to press. In particular, Grace Hong connected us to Richard Morrison at Fordham and has been a tireless supporter and mentor on this project from the moment Jacob arrived at UCLA. The UCLA Center for the Study of Women and former Gender Studies Chair Chris Littleton provided much-needed research grants that allowed Jacob to travel to Harvard and complete this project with Cameron during the summer of 2010. Eleanor Craig and Toby Oldham gave Jacob a warm home to come back to during that time and since the beginning of this journey. Jacob would also like to thank his Gender Studies colleagues and mentors who have provided feedback and lent various forms of support to this project in its several stages, in particular: Freda Fair, Morgan Woolsey, Jessica Martinez, Naveen Minai, Jocelyn Thomas, Dalal Alfares, Aren Aizura, and Rachel Lee. He is thankful for the various Laus who may not have known exactly what he was working on but were nonetheless excited. Last but certainly not least, to his twin Amy for seeing Jacob through it all.

We both would very much like to thank the team at Fordham University Press, particularly Richard Morrison, who has been such an enthusiastic supporter of this project. Fordham's anonymous reviewers also offered valuable, constructive feedback, for which we sincerely thank them. We are very grateful for Susan Stryker's generous support, both in writing the Foreword and in encouraging both of us over our years of work on this project.

Finally, we want to acknowledge Michael Dillon/Lobzang Jivaka, a man of our grandparents' generation, whose writings have helped open pathways to many in the trans community. We come to the completion of this project with gratitude for his willingness to share his journey with those who have come after him and hope that the publication of his narrative will do that justice.